PRAISE FOR *OUT OF THE BOX*

'In this engaging book, we hear directly from the true experts — autistic people and their families — and how we, as a community, can best support their lives. A treat to read.' — **Andrew Whitehouse, Professor of Autism Research and Director of CliniKids at the Telethon Kids Institute**

'Understanding neurodiversity, including autism and ADHD, has become essential for our community's progress. *Out of the Box* will be hugely helpful to parents and family members, teachers, health professionals, politicians, and policy-makers. I highly recommend it for its breadth and depth.' — **Dr Michelle Garnett, Clinical Psychologist – PhD (Psych), Co-founder and Director of Attwood & Garnett Events, AuDHD**

'A brilliant piece of work, revealing an astonishing amount of research into the joys and challenges of neurodiversity. *Out of the Box* celebrates different ways of thinking and behaving as part of the rich tapestry of life. It maps a clear path ahead for researchers, educators, and carers. This book should be in every school library.' — **Tracey Spicer, journalist and author**

'Your child will thank you for reading this book.' — **Sally Hepworth, author**

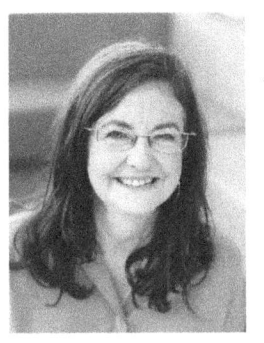

Madonna King is an award-winning journalist and author, whose understanding of teenage lives is valued through speaking and writing engagements across the nation. As a journalist and commentator, she continues to work across TV, radio and online, and all her books are based on hundreds of expert interviews. Her bestselling parenting books give a voice to tweens and teens aged 8–18 and include *Ten-Ager, Being 14, Fathers and Daughters, L Platers* and *Saving our Kids*. Madonna travels Australia, talking to school communities and students about the challenges that mark their teen years. Learn more at madonnaking.com.au.

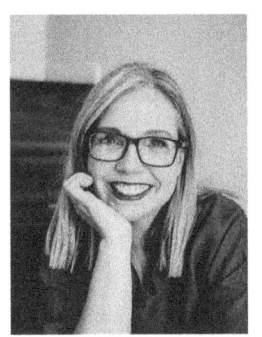

Rebecca Sparrow is a teen educator, the author of six books and the host of ABC's *Parental As Anything, Teens* podcast. Each year, Bec speaks to thousands of tweens and teens (and their parents) about how to recognise and nurture strong friendships, navigate conflict and set healthy boundaries. Her online friendship webinars are watched in lounge rooms across the world. Bec is also an ambassador for The Lady Musgrave Trust, which provides support and services to young women facing homelessness. Learn more at rebeccasparrow.com.

First published 2024 by University of Queensland Press
PO Box 6042, St Lucia, Queensland 4067 Australia

University of Queensland Press (UQP) acknowledges the Traditional Owners and their custodianship of the lands on which UQP operates. We pay our respects to their Ancestors and their descendants, who continue cultural and spiritual connections to Country. We recognise their valuable contributions to Australian and global society.

uqp.com.au
reception@uqp.com.au

Copyright © Madonna King and Rebecca Sparrow 2024
The moral rights of the authors have been asserted.

This book is copyright. Except for private study, research, criticism or reviews, as permitted under the *Copyright Act*, no part of this book may be reproduced, stored in a retrieval system, or transmitted in any form or by any means without prior written permission. Enquiries should be made to the publisher.

Cover design by Christa Moffitt / Christabella Designs
Cover photograph by Pasuwan/Shutterstock
Typeset in 12/16 pt Bembo Std and 10.5/16 pt Trade Gothic Next Ltd by
Post Pre-press Group, Brisbane
Printed in Australia by McPherson's Printing Group

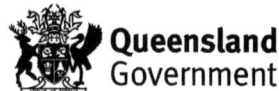 University of Queensland Press is supported by the Queensland Government through Arts Queensland.

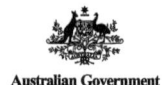 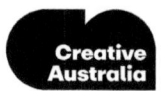 University of Queensland Press is assisted by the Australian Government through Creative Australia, its principal arts investment and advisory body.

A catalogue record for this book is available from the National Library of Australia.

ISBN 978 0 7022 6877 9 (pbk)
ISBN 978 0 7022 7014 7 (epdf)
ISBN 978 0 7022 7015 4 (epub)

University of Queensland Press uses papers that are natural, renewable and recyclable products made from wood grown in well-managed forests and other controlled sources. The logging and manufacturing processes conform to the environmental regulations of the country of origin.

Madonna King and
Rebecca Sparrow

Out of the Box

UQP

CONTENTS

Glossary   ix
A Note on Language   xv
Introduction: The Starting Line   1
1. Diagnosis, Labels and Language   9

PART I: FRIENDSHIPS   33
2. Friendships in Primary School   35
3. Friendships in High School   52
4. Schoolyard Dynamics   73

PART II: EDUCATION   85
5. Finding the Right School   87
6. The Power of a Teacher   106
7. To the Principal's Office   124
8. From the Teacher's Desk   141

PART III: SPREADING YOUR WINGS   159
9. Join a Club and Get the Golden Ticket   161
10. A Family Affair   172
11. Life After School   187
12. Dating and Driving   210

PART IV: THE FUTURE LOOKS BRIGHT   223
13. NDIS and the New Landscape   225
14. Research and the Way Ahead   238

Resources   252
Acknowledgements   274
Index   277

GLOSSARY

The following glossary is not an exhaustive list, but a starting point to describe some of the conditions discussed in this book. Many of these terms are changing over time with input from the neuro-affirming community.

ASPERGER SYNDROME or ASPERGER'S is a developmental condition; the term was formerly used to denote a diagnosis on the autism spectrum. It affects how people behave and deal with others. Asperger Syndrome is considered a high-function form of autism.

ATTENTION DEFICIT DISORDER (ADD) is an outdated term that has been used for the inattentive type of ADHD without characteristics of hyperactivity.

ATTENTION DEFICIT HYPERACTIVITY DISORDER (ADHD) is a developmental difference that can cause problems with concentration, focus, hyperactivity and impulsivity. It affects the brain's executive functioning, and a person's capacity to self-regulate their thoughts and emotions. Boys are often diagnosed earlier than girls, many of whom 'mask' their condition. ADHD can present in three ways: inattentive symptoms, hyperactive-impulsive symptoms or a combination of those. ADHD is routinely treated with medicine.

AUTISM is a neurodevelopmental condition where people differ in how they communicate and interact socially; some might be highly focused or have sensory sensitivities. Autism was formerly widely known as Autism Spectrum Disorder (ASD), indicating the range of differences between autistic people. While autism presents challenges, it can also deliver unique skills and capabilities. Often, autism presents with other conditions.

CHILDHOOD DISINTEGRATIVE DISORDER (CDD) was first documented by Theodor Heller in 1908. The disorder is characterised by a loss of acquired language, motor and social skills after a period of normal development to at least the age of two. CDD is rare.

DIAGNOSTIC OVERSHADOWING occurs when a health professional wrongly assumes that symptoms being presented to them are a direct consequence of a patient's disability or co-existing mental health condition, rather than considering or exploring alternatives.

DOUBLE EMPATHY PROBLEM is a theory first coined by sociologist and social psychologist Damian Milton in 2012. It suggests when people of very different experiences interact — such as an autistic and a non-autistic person — they can find it challenging to empathise with each other. It is a 'double' problem because both people experience it.

DYSCALCULIA impacts an individual's ability to do mathematics and is characterised by inability to see, handle and understand numbers. According to the Australian Dyslexia Association, experts don't yet

GLOSSARY

know for sure if dyscalculia is more common in girls or in boys, but most agree it's unlikely that there's any significant difference.

DYSLEXIA is a brain-based difference characterised by difficulties with reading and spelling despite having the ability to learn. Dyslexia occurs on a spectrum from mild to severe.

DYSPRAXIA is a neurological condition, which is also called Developmental Coordination Disorder (DCD). More often identified in boys, a child with dyspraxia might struggle with gross and fine motor skills. A lifelong condition, it affects about one in twenty children.

GLASS CHILD/CHILDREN is a term used to describe how siblings of a neurodivergent (ND) child can feel when their parents' focus and energy is not equally directed at them; they say they feel 'invisible' next to the struggles of their sibling.

MASKING describes when people hide or camouflage neurodivergent traits to 'fit in' with their peer group. This is most often seen in women and girls, who can be older at the time of first diagnosis.

NATIONAL DISABILITY INSURANCE SCHEME (NDIS) is run by the Commonwealth Government to provide funding support for people with disabilities. It was legislated in 2013, before a national rollout in 2020. It aims to provide those with a disability more independence, better access to skills and jobs, or to enhance their quality of life. The NDIS is run by the National Disability Insurance Agency (NDIA).

NEURODIVERGENT (ND) is a non-medical term that refers to a person or a group of people whose brains are 'wired' differently and who are not considered neurotypical (NT). A person is ND when they have a diagnosed neuro-processing difference. Many conditions fall under the neurodivergence category, including autism, ADHD, dyslexia and Tourette Syndrome, and are often co-occuring.

NEURODIVERSITY refers to the diversity of all human brains, and the different ways in which we interact with the world; there is no correct or single way to think, learn or behave. These behavioural traits are regarded as part of normal variation in the human population, where 'different' does not mean 'deficit'.

NEUROTYPICAL (NT) refers to people who conform to typical norms of neurological functioning. This term is used for someone who is not neurodivergent.

OPPOSITIONAL DEFIANT DISORDER (ODD) is a childhood behaviour disorder where children frequently refuse to do what others ask them to do, especially if they're tired, upset or frustrated. According to the Raising Children Network, while this characteristic can be seen in all children at times, kids with ODD behave like this a lot and it interferes with their ability to learn and communicate, manage emotions and get along with others. ODD often begins during the preschool years.

PATHOLOGICAL DEMAND AVOIDANCE (PDA) is a condition associated with autism. It is not common but is characterised by an overwhelming or obsessional need to resist demands by refusing, withdrawing or ignoring them. This can lead to both meltdowns and violent outbursts. PDA can deliver strong anxiety where a person feels like they have lost control, which can feel like a panic attack.

PERVASIVE DEVELOPMENTAL DISORDER (PDD) is characterised by delays in the development of social and communication skills,

GLOSSARY

including: language; relating to people and events; playing with toys and other objects; and dealing with a change in environment or routine. It can include repetitive body movements or behaviour patterns.

SCHOOL REFUSAL is when high levels of distress and a reluctance to attend class can cause an increase in non-attendance. It is not the same as truancy. Many experts believe 'refusal' is the wrong word, suggesting that 'school can't' is a more accurate term to describe a child's reluctance to go to school.

STIMMING is a behaviour that some autistic people engage in and can include various actions, including: rocking; hand-flapping; posturing; chewing; listening to the same noise over and over again; or engaging in repetitive physical movements, such as flicking a switch on and off. Stimming varies between children and is thought to help them cope with both strong emotions and sensory information.

THEORY OF MIND is a psychological term that refers to the ability to understand that other people have different beliefs, views, intentions and emotions from our own.

TOURETTE SYNDROME (TS) is characterised by rapid, repetitive and involuntary muscle movements and vocalisations called 'tics', and often involves behavioural difficulties. According to the Tourette Syndrome Association of Australia, tics are experienced as a build-up of tension, are irresistible and eventually must be performed. Typically tics increase as a result of tension or stress and decrease with relaxation or concentration on an absorbing task.

A NOTE ON LANGUAGE

For consistency, in this book we have adopted identity-first language to reflect the majority preference of the neurodivergent community we spoke to. They often reject person-first language, because it attempts to separate neurodiverse people from their neurotype and follows a medical model of disability, rather than a social model. People who look at autism through a medical model lens view it with a focus on diagnosing autism and co-conditions as a disability. People who look at autism through a social model lens see it as a neurological difference that should be accommodated, and believe that autistic behaviours should be better understood and socially accepted.

While the definition pendulum is swinging away from the medical model, it is important to note that these black-and-white definitions can vary for people across the spectrum. Some characteristics of autism can make life difficult for the person receiving support and therefore funding for these aspects, as recognised by the medical model, is critical. At the same time, other characteristics of autism can be the source of success, pleasure, connection and achievement. Embracing a strengths-based social model is crucial for adaptive functioning and quality of life.

INTRODUCTION: THE STARTING LINE

MOLLY, SEVENTEEN, IS DIRECT WHEN asked about her biggest daily challenge. 'Life,' she says. Why? 'Because the world isn't made for people like me.'

Molly is autistic and was diagnosed at the age of fifteen, more than a decade after her parents noticed milestone differences between their toddler daughter and her siblings. 'Until her mental health fell off a cliff,' Molly's mother says, 'outside of the house she didn't often look like someone who needed help.' That made it difficult for Molly and her family to access, or even to know how to ask for, help.

Molly's teachers and peers assumed that because she was passing her subjects and seemed to fit in, she was managing as well as any other teenager. But every day, trying to do what others took for granted, became what her mother termed an 'invisible struggle'. 'She masks so well that people can forget she is autistic, so when she slips up, she's treated as if she is making excuses. The way she experiences life is invalidated daily at school.'

Molly isn't alone. The teachers we spoke to during our research for this book said that between ten and forty per cent of their classes were often made up of neurodivergent (ND) students. While their ages may differ, with some just toddlers while others are driving, dating, studying or working, these people share a bond – their neurodivergence makes them different in a world that values those who are neurotypical (NT).

Autistic children (and adults) have a different brain to NT people, and one byproduct of that is that they don't always intuitively understand other people's emotions. That means reading facial expressions and body language, or perceiving what someone might be thinking, can be challenging. There are other differences, too – some autistic people find change difficult and can experience sensory overload. But, like all of us, every autistic person is unique: 'If you've met one person with autism, you've met one person with autism,' is a quote made famous by autistic professor Dr Stephen Shore who works to improve the potential of those on the autism spectrum.

> *'When I think of how hard my days are advocating for my kids, I need to remind myself how hard it is for them in a world that doesn't accept them. They are the ones trying to change things for future generations, and it's so difficult.'*

Attention Deficit Hyperactivity Disorder (ADHD) is another condition that sits under the ND umbrella. It can show up as inattention in young children, who may also be easily distracted and impulsive. Under-diagnosed in girls, an ADHD diagnosis is more common than autism, with estimates of one in twenty Australians believed to have ADHD.

There are many other conditions that fall under an ND label. Dyslexia is a condition that involves people experiencing difficulties in writing and spelling. Dyspraxia involves challenges around motor skills. Dyscalculia involves challenges with numbers. Tourette Syndrome causes involuntary physical and vocal 'tics', while people with Oppositional Defiant Disorder (ODD) present with symptoms of anger and irritability, such as persistent arguing.

Disappointingly, autism and ADHD both include the word 'disorder' in their title. However, expert advice within the ND community asserts that while neurodivergence may be a disability in many cases, it is not a 'disorder'; a point made clear by the fact that ND people range from intellectually impaired, non-speaking, socially challenged through to intellectually gifted. Our research confirmed this to be true: while we heard many stories full of heartache, there were also many stories of courage, connection, triumph and joy.

> *'I'm lonely because my brain is different to everyone else, and I think differently.'*

Like the discrimination meted out to groups based on ethnicity or gender, ND children are too often left stage-side, waiting for their place in the limelight; a place they have to fight much harder to win. That fight starts before diagnosis and can last a lifetime. Sometimes it's due to the challenges their condition brings, but often it is because of the battles they face in accessing funding, education and employment, and finding friendships. Often, they are judged harshly by peers and the parents of peers who lack an understanding of ND behaviours. In communities and schools that promote inclusion, ND kids are missing out on opportunities and critical emotional support in their formative years. As one parent explained: 'I wish people understood that autism is not a deficit. It is a difference, and that difference comes with challenges, but it also comes with a different way of seeing things and questioning things, which I think is wonderful.'

This book belongs to autistic and ADHD kids: their path to achievement could be made so much easier if everyone just listened to their voices. Our world is made up of remarkable ND minds that have changed the course of history – across science and literature, comedy and education. Learning from our ND community can provide other opportunities for our education system and our workplaces; built environments that, if tweaked, could unlock a phenomenal resource.

The ongoing research of scientists across the world should give us enormous hope. With this book, we want to help turn up the volume on those voices, which have been muted too often in history. We want everyone to listen to the parents who are advocating for ND kids, the health professionals who spend their waking hours in clinics dispensing expert advice, the scientists who are exploring the future, and the schoolteachers who spend their days devoted to educating the next generation.

Our goal is to help ND children take their place in classrooms and workplaces, and for NT children, parents, teachers and employers to understand the invisible challenges and untapped potential of those sitting beside them. ND children don't need to prove their worth. As human beings they have every right to be valued for who they are.

As part of the research for this book, we surveyed 1300 families who have an immediate family member, mostly children, who identify as neurodivergent. The focus of our survey was to probe parents – and willing children – about their diagnosis, the challenges they confronted, and the obstacles and opportunities they've experienced along the way. We also asked them to nominate the resources that have helped them, and used their wisdom to compile a wealth of useful resources for families and educators – from austism and ADHD experts, parenting organisations and online learning resources, to books on neurodiversity for primary and high school-aged kids.

Some of the families we surveyed had multiple ND children; in others, parents also had their own ND diagnosis. To understand what is needed to help our children thrive, we looked specifically at their interactions with teachers and the education system, how they developed and sustained friendships, and how they navigated life after school, including work, driving and intimate relationships.

Once significant trends emerged, we then interviewed dozens of those families and sought the advice of almost 600 educators about the ND children in their classrooms, their interaction with parents, the current curriculum, classroom set-up, and their own training in this area. With that information, provided by almost 2000 people, we sought out global experts, many of whom are also autistic or have ADHD. Their advice is directed at parents, who daily support the ND children in their lives, and the educators who welcome them into their classrooms each day.

THE VALUE OF DIFFERENCE

Myths about neurodivergence can spread like a bad contagion across classrooms and within communities and, as a result, influence policymaking. Aidan, a Year 8 autistic student, tackled this issue in a class assignment, telling his peers: 'I hope you learn something.' He then clinically turned his attention to their prevailing views, to demolish myths that many still believe, including, 'everyone in the world is at least a little bit autistic'. This is what he said:

MYTH: 'People who don't look autistic aren't autistic.'

REALITY: 'This is completely false. For some people who are on the autism spectrum, it's obvious, but for other people, it's not as obvious.'

MYTH: 'Autism can be cured.'

REALITY: 'There is no cure for autism, as (again) it is not a disease or illness. Instead, you can help and support people with autism to feel more comfortable in their surroundings. One of the best ways to help is to learn more about autism so the autistic person feels safe and comfortable around you.'

Aidan says he was prompted to do the assignment because, 'a lot of the class used autism as an insult … and that sort of told me that they didn't know what they were talking about'.

As our research indicated, many autistic people view the idea of being 'cured' as offensive. They believe that we should stop seeing neurodivergence as a medical condition and treat it as a part of the rich tapestry of life. We support this thinking strongly. This book aims to dispel some of the common misconceptions about autism and ADHD, so that we all – ND and NT – can better understand each other and appreciate the value of difference.

LET'S DISPEL SOME MYTHS

In their own voices, the ND community shared with us real-life experiences of some of the misinformation often heard floating around the schoolyard and in the wider community. This is what they told us:

MYTH: All ND people are the same.
REALITY: 'Different is beautiful! Some of the most talented and famous people – artists, authors, celebrities, chefs and surgeons – are ND. Never let that stop you from being happy and successful … just find a different path there.'

MYTH: ADHD presents the same way in boys and girls.
REALITY: 'Boys in my class were singled out in primary school. I was at university before my ADHD was diagnosed. Boys and girls are very different, and girls hide or mask it because we don't want to be different, I guess.'

MYTH: Autistic people don't have a sense of humour.
REALITY: 'My twelve-year-old autistic son has flourished in upper primary because of his fabulous sense of humour. Making the class (and his teacher) laugh has helped him feel good about going to school and made him a valued member of the class because, as one classmate said in a Christmas card last year: *Thanks for making us crack-up laughing. Our class would have been boring without you.*'

MYTH: Autistic kids are unemotional.
REALITY: 'My boy is so emotional but he tries to hide or mask it, so no one knows he is different.'

MYTH: Kids on the spectrum are all good at maths.
REALITY: '[My son] is very aware of things other kids excel at – he knows who gets their spelling words right, who gets picked first for games, who gets awards that are "real" and not because it's "just their turn so it looks fair" … He is also very aware that he cannot identify any one thing that he considers himself to be good at, because "stuff is hard for me".'

MYTH: ADHD is an excuse for naughty behaviour.
REALITY: 'I'm trying to do what teachers want me to do. Being at school, I didn't really know what was required of me. If I asked [the] teachers [they] just said I was not listening or being naughty, but each teacher had different rules. All the kids and teachers think I'm a bad kid, and everyone ... is watching me and waiting for me to be bad.'

MYTH: Autistic children cannot hold eye contact or be social.
REALITY: 'My daughter can participate in a social conversation, as good as the next person, with perfect eye contact. That's one thing that made her diagnosis difficult.'

MYTH: Non-speaking means non-thinking.
REALITY: 'My son cannot speak, but he can read, identify classical composers and count. He keenly observes everything around him and is too smart for his own good!'

MYTH: Most autistic children are gifted at something.
REALITY: 'I mean, it's a nice idea, but replacing a negative bias with a positive bias is still a bias. And I find it really demoralising constantly looking for a "gift". Most normal kids don't have gifts – why am I expecting him to develop one?'

MYTH: ADHD is a result of bad parenting, or caused by exposure to technology.
REALITY: 'Every parent of a ND child is already blaming themselves either because of red flags or early signs we just didn't pick up, or because we lose our temper and our patience with our kids. Having other parents judging us when our kids are melting down or stimming brings a huge amount of shame to the whole experience.'

1. DIAGNOSIS, LABELS AND LANGUAGE

'Love is blind.' That's Professor Tony Attwood's answer when asked what he learnt about himself after he discovered his son, Will, was autistic. Attwood is a global expert in autism, a clinical psychologist with decades of experience, as well as a best-selling author whose books have been published in dozens of languages. But despite his expertise, and diagnosing an untold number of autistic children, it took him three decades to realise his own son, who struggled with drug addiction, was autistic. His answer shows a hint, perhaps, of how he might have remonstrated with himself over that delay; that he didn't see that his own son, from early on, had shown autistic traits. But it also shows, with startling clarity, how a diagnosis of autism can be mired in confusion and doubt, and disbelief.

Dr Bronwyn Sutton, a speech pathologist at Sutton Speech, has an autistic son and says there is a very simple explanation for why parents often don't pick up on neurodivergence in their child. 'The answer is love. We are supposed to look at our children through rose-coloured glasses.'

Attwood's personal story, like thousands of others, points to how tricky a diagnosis can be. Although, as many parents and experts told us along the way, the diagnosis can be the easy part; it's what to do next that can present bigger challenges.

EARLY SIGNS

Early signs of neurodivergence – whether autism, ADHD or another condition – are not the same for everyone. Plenty of parents have dismissed some of the key traits, such as a delightful quirkiness or a formidable energy, that later resulted in a diagnosis. But to make things even more confusing, many neurotypical children also share these traits. The age when it might become clear that a child needs support can also vary widely. More often than not, an autistic child will have co-occurring conditions, and sometimes this provides the impetus for seeking a diagnosis.

So, what should we – as parents, grandparents and carers – look for in a child to detect early signs of neurodivergence? How do we obtain a diagnosis or assessment? What will it mean for our child? And for our family? The questions are endless, and the answers are not always what parents want to hear. Some parents want to 'cure' a child or take back a diagnosis so that their child will not have to wear a 'label'. They grieve for the child they thought they'd have, not the treasured one in front of them, who is likely to turn their whole life, and the life of those around them, upside down.

For Attwood, the signs his son was autistic were always there, but it wasn't until he was watching an old family movie of them together at the ocean's edge, that the penny finally dropped. Will was in his own world, not engaging with his father or seeking out the hand in front of him. Just a tiny slice in time, decades earlier, provided answers to so much that has happened since. (Will was later diagnosed with autism Level 1, formerly known as Asperger's). The telltale signs of neurodivergence can be mixed and unclear, and that's because, as Attwood says, autism usually comes 'with friends', such as ADHD, anxiety, depression and a host of other conditions. In our research, this also stood out – eating disorders among autistic tween and teen girls are common, as are the number of autistic teens who are questioning their gender. These co-existing conditions can make it more difficult for parents to identify, especially when making comparisons with a peer group as they reach expected milestones. Is she just 'off with the fairies' or does her creative imagination signal something else?

So broad are the early signs of autism, that many parents – particularly with a first child – doubt themselves. As one mother explained: 'There is so much rubbish that people say that means nothing; advice people give because they think they're trying to reassure you that you're being a good parent, instead of actually listening to your challenges and taking them seriously.'

Parents and teachers told us they would hear many classic excuses for a child's behaviour, such as, 'he's just being a boy'; 'boys can't sit still'; 'boys are messy'; 'boys are noisy'.

'When she started Year 7, she had major trouble regulating her emotions – big meltdowns.'

In our survey, the early signs of neurodivergence were commonly noticed during early school years or in the transition to high school, when students receive heavier workloads while at the same time experience less structure and routine. During Covid lockdowns, when children were unable to attend school, many parents noticed their child's behaviours first-hand – an inability to focus or sit still, taking forever to do a task, or having a meltdown. In the case of ADHD, young women are frequently diagnosed in their first or second year at university.

When we asked parents what they noticed as the first indicator they had a neurodivergent child, they told us the signs were mixed, confusing and varied. They included: sleep and food issues; delayed milestones (particularly with language); being anxious; expressing sensory challenges; having meltdowns; missing social cues; not following simple instructions and being unable to complete more than two steps of a direction at a time. As one parent explained, there can be many mixed signals, which on their own don't add up to much, but together paint a different picture. 'In Prep and on play dates I noticed he wasn't playing with his friends. He was off in his own imaginary world playing a game by himself. He would cry if a teacher called on him to answer a question on the spot – frozen with the stress of having to answer. He had increasing anxiety over heights even on play equipment. The phrases "quick sticks" or "hurry up" would send him over the edge. A year later we noticed he couldn't join in any after-school sporting experiences, like little kids' soccer or AFL, with all his mates. He couldn't follow verbal instructions from the coaches and then would cry. And he couldn't detect sarcasm and took everything literally.'

Parents described many others telltale traits across childhood, including: always being busy; school refusal; separation anxiety; stimming; being chaotic and disorganised; lacking time awareness. Ritualistic behaviours, such as chewing on clothes or lining up toys, or only playing with particular colours or shapes, were also noticeable. ND kids also tend to have distinct characteristics: they might be a rule follower, a change-disliker, a fidgeter, have a lack of impulse control or an inflated sense of social justice. Some have difficulty in making, and keeping, friends. They might appear to be disengaged, talk excessively, have learning difficulties, or display difficult behaviours – often ending up with them being regularly disciplined or suspended from school.

> '[Our son] had the speed and energy of a thousand men.'

Because every child is different, the age when they are diagnosed can also vary widely. In our survey, it ranged from the age of three years right through to adulthood. Here, in their own words, parents describe the first time they noticed that their child was different:

- 'I was helping in his class and noticed he behaved in quite an antisocial manner, and his peers were reacting negatively.'
- 'First indicator: an interest in road maps and street directions.'
- 'Anxiety at two; fussy eater as a toddler; severe sleep dysregulation from baby to childhood; separation anxiety at kindy.'
- 'Struggling to multitask at high school when demands became greater; poor self-esteem.'
- 'He was very clingy as a three-year-old. It was initially put down to anxiety, until we saw a GP who had personal experience and who asked more questions. We realised he didn't make eye contact, didn't do any imaginative play, didn't answer to his name.'
- 'When she was a toddler, she would only pick up and play with yellow balls in a ball pit. This went on for a year and then it changed to blue.'

- 'Discovered when she was fifteen. First indicator: not handing in schoolwork. Until then she appeared like any other child.'

For girls in their mid-teens, parents often realised there was an issue when their daughters were 'not completing work' or 'not handing in schoolwork'. Some young women were diagnosed at university, when routines changed. In several of those cases, symptoms of anxiety or depression were the impetus for seeking help. Some ND girls became more aware of their behaviours through the social media stories of peers, particularly on TikTok.

> **'She's always been my firecracker. But the older she got the less I could excuse her outbursts.'**

Dr Tamara Rosier, founder of the ADHD Center of West Michigan in the US, has also served as president of the ADHD Coaches Organization and is the author of *Your Brain's Not Broken*. She raises the issue for young adult women who only discover their condition once the structures of school and home disappear.

'A lot of us with ADHD, we feel sad and lonely and ashamed all the time because we're not meeting people's expectations. And so that's very unfortunate. And that's really hard for us. So, if you can see yourself and go, "wait a minute, maybe I'm not broken. Maybe my brain's just different", well, that's good.' But, she says navigating the tricky second step in this thinking is also important. 'Let's just not fly the flag that "I'm different". Let's figure out strategies so that I can do what I want to do in life.' No one deserves to miss that second step.

DIAGNOSIS, LABELS AND LANGUAGE

Autism expert and clinical psychologist Dr Michelle Garnett specialised in autism for thirty years before seeking external validation for what she had suspected to be true for seven years. Before being late diagnosed as autistic and having ADHD, Garnett, like many who camouflage, understood her own struggles were due to social anxiety and depression. She worried about being stigmatised, but was inspired by two ADHD clinical psychologists – Monique Mitchelson and Mandy Hansen – and sought a diagnosis to feel confident to be 'out'. Garnett says: 'I wanted to be part of the ND-affirming movement that says it is not only okay to be ND, it is possible to be strong, successful and influential with ND.' She goes on to say: 'Also, it became much safer to be out. Prior to that, I didn't feel safe that it would be received in the way it should. I knew what it meant but I didn't believe others would.'

When a parent pushes for an assessment for their child – and some push for years – often it starts with a niggling gut instinct that keeps them awake at night and asking questions during the day. 'With our daughter, we just had the feeling in the back of our minds for several years.' Another said: 'There was no one thing, it was a series of things – observations, comments by educators and other family members. I had a moment this year where I suddenly thought, in so many ways I think my son is trying his best, perhaps he is genuinely trying his best to focus and pay attention but actually … can't. I realised, then, that I would trust my gut and get him some help and understanding.'

As speech pathologist Bronwyn Sutton says, love can blur clarity, and in many cases, it can be someone else who taps a parent on the shoulder and suggests further investigation. The gentle guidance of early teachers here looms large. Teachers and educators are able to compare children in the classroom and identify who needs support with various tasks. 'Year 1 teacher suggested an assessment based on symptoms,' said one parent. 'School didn't see a problem, but his tutor suggested testing,' said another.

> *'I had no idea what ADHD was. I used to call her an airhead. Her Year 3 teacher suggested there may be a problem.'*

While interventions by educators of this nature are not always welcome, many parents are grateful that the differences in their child are not being overlooked. They found it confirmed their own doubts and was the impetus for them seeking a diagnosis: 'Teacher suggested there was something going on in Prep due to her lack of empathy. We had no idea.' Another parent admitted: 'Gentle nudges from excellent teachers. Up until then I thought I was an inadequate parent.'

Sutton asks parents to consider the motives of a teacher who raises a challenge for their child. 'The only reason a teacher would say anything about your child is from a place of care. They're not doing it for any other reason, except that they care for the child,' she says.

Asked about the early signs of autism that stand out to her, Sutton explains that autistic children often see 'people as hard and sameness as good'. That 'lack of connection' with others can be one of the first concrete signs. 'I would say that being autistic means that connecting with other people, particularly peers, is really tricky,' she says.

In early childhood, where groups of children are playing, these behaviours sometimes stand out. So can a 'passionate love of sameness' or not liking change. 'From the ages of one to six, children are going through massive change – what they eat, where they sleep, toileting, everything. So that challenge with constant change is usually an early sign.' Resistance to change might manifest itself in tears or even meltdowns. 'But for some children, particularly girls, that distress might be projected inwardly, and it might appear as shutting down, not talking, not communicating.'

Many parents told us that delayed speech was also a developmental marker that prompted them to seek advice. Sutton said that speech pathologists often see this in children in the lead-up to an official diagnosis.

SEEKING HELP

Getting a diagnosis is much more complex than a trip to the family doctor. Indeed, different conditions involve a range of assessments, and almost always include a paediatrician if the child is aged under eighteen, or a psychiatrist if the diagnosis is being sought by a young adult. But while a paediatrician or psychiatrist might deliver the official diagnosis required to unlock and access support, including government funding, other professionals play a key role. For example, a visit to an occupational therapist (OT), speech pathologist or psychologist might prompt the initial consideration of an assessment. A GP is important in ruling out other conditions and will also likely know the family – and a child's – history. They can make referrals to specialists, who in turn can determine the level of support required.

Victorian paediatrician Dr Mandira Hiremath specialises in autism assessments. While non-binding, she says gold-standard national guidelines exist for both autism and ADHD. Hiremath, who has two autistic children, says those guidelines take a step back from medical diagnosis and towards a support-based diagnosis: finding out what assistance a child or adult might need.

Hiremath supports a three-pronged approach to diagnosis. The first step involves a medical assessment of the needs of the child, including an overview of their background to better understand genetic and environmental markers in their lives. This is crucial, she says, because other factors like trauma or adverse child experiences might sometimes mirror the signs of autism. The second part of the approach is seeking multidisciplinary input from other health providers, including speech and occupational therapists, as well as psychologists. The third and final part of the diagnosis involves 'checking in' with parents to explain the assessment, and to see how it sits with their understanding of their child.

Professor Andrew Whitehouse, a global expert in autism, says while national guidelines exist, clinicians have to 'work within the system'. His comments allude to the delays experienced by many families in seeking assessment and diagnosis. But all things being equal, he relies on 'a multidisciplinary team comprising of a paediatrician, speech pathologist and psychologist who observe the behaviours of the child – because while autism is very much a genetically-based condition … we diagnose on what we can see.' This might include, for example, social communication difficulties or strict and repetitive behaviours. 'A clinical team observes the child in a range of different settings and seeks to understand whether that child chose those behaviours or if there is any other explanation for those behaviours, and if there's not, that's when a diagnosis is made.'

Sutton says that the diagnostic process can often start early with a speech therapist or OT. This is important, because often when a child doesn't meet milestones a speech therapist or OT might be the first port of call for a parent. Sutton says an OT might consider the child's ability to regulate their emotions, for example, and will consider the child's social communication and ability to communicate with peers. Depending on age and need, the child might also be visiting a psychologist. This is particularly the case with tweens and teens. Once armed with all the information, a family could visit their GP and the child might then be referred to a paediatrician who has the professional advice of that team – including an OT and/or speech therapist – in front of them, ahead of making a diagnosis. With a young adult, the process might be more direct – going from a psychologist or a GP, who might then refer them to a psychiatrist. It's a similar process for ADHD and other conditions.

Sydney GP and former president of the Australian Medical Association (NSW) Dr Michael Bonning says autism and ADHD are the most common forms of neurodivergence in most GP clinics. He sees the apparent rise in numbers as a product of increased awareness, and is critical of suggestions that NDIS government funding has created a higher number of diagnoses, saying the rise predates its existence. He agrees that a regular family GP is invaluable in identifying signs of neurodivergence. 'One of the things that GPs pick up on, is we know our patients for a long time. Women and high achievers, especially, are often overlooked or misdiagnosed because they don't necessarily display those hallmark disruptive behaviours in childhood.'

When asked what a parent should tell a GP if they are concerned about their child, Bonning urges them to simply tell a story and explain the context of their concern. What did they see? How did their child react? He says this will prompt a GP to ask more questions – because every child is different. He provides the example of an elderly patient who has lost their life partner to illustrate his point. They might turn up for an appointment, dressed impeccably, and sound like 'they've got everything together'. But a home visit, or a discussion with their children, might paint a very different picture, and this can unlock support and assistance that allows them to remain in their own home. 'The more you can tell your GP, the better,' Bonning says. He urges parents to also ensure they understand the next steps in the process towards diagnosis, before leaving an appointment.

Attwood says science hasn't delivered all the answers around autism and its causes. 'All I can say is, for the majority of autistic children, the apple doesn't fall far from the tree.' When a child is diagnosed, often someone else in the family – parents, aunts or grandparents – will also have similar traits. It is not unusual to have more than one autistic child.

Furthermore, in eighty-five per cent of diagnoses autism co-exists or co-occurs with other conditions, such as ADHD, anxiety and depression. For many adults, Attwood believes it is not autism that provides the biggest challenge, but anxiety or depression, particularly when it comes to employment.

'Research and my own clinical experience suggest that around one in four patients with an eating disorder, substance abuse, gender dysphoria or borderline personality disorder have a dual diagnosis. There is also an association between autism and Tourette Syndrome, sleep disorders and bipolar disorders.'

Complexities arise because every individual is different; with autism there is no one-size-fits-all explanation. For example, pathological demand avoidance (PDA) was first identified in the 1980s but has become increasingly more common. It's described as a very high anxiety where the individual needs to both control and avoid other people's expectations and demands. Attwood says it is considered as an atypical type of autism but differs from 'typical autism in that the person shows a superficial sociability and capacity to read situations to the extent that they can manipulate them to avoid complying with demands.' As Attwood recognises, 'Unfortunately, the strategies frequently used [to manage] autism are often ineffective and counterproductive for a child with a PDA profile.'

Puberty is also a concerning time when autism can present new problems. Attwood believes about one-third of autistic teens go through puberty without any change in their condition. 'A third will have a deterioration in concentration – we say the brain is closed for renovation,' although it returns a couple of years later. But, for one in three, it can be devastating. In those cases, major psychological issues – eating disorders, self-harm and depression – can result. While almost all teens embark on a process of self-identity, autistic teens often ponder such questions 'at a depth and intensity more than others'.

MEDICATION AND THERAPY

Once a diagnosis is made, a team of professional consultants is crucial to a child's long-term success. While a specialist might provide a formal diagnosis and unlock support, therapists, a psychologist and a range of other professionals can be crucial in helping a child reach their full potential. For example, some families have employed a music therapist or embarked on art or equine therapy.

Clinical psychologist Dr Wesley Turner says a psychologist is able to help people become 'attuned to themselves and attuned to the world and the people around them'. He says that's just as important in an adult diagnosis because people might have adopted coping mechanisms that are not ideal. He gives the example of teen girls not establishing boundaries or speaking up for themselves. 'I cut my teeth learning how to diagnose and treat young teenage women, which was a wonderful experience,' he says. 'But for a variety of reasons, they haven't been able to trust their gut reaction. So, a lot of what we're doing is undoing the unhelpful coping patterns that they've learnt.'

So, where does a pharmacist sit here, in a child's support team? Yvette Anderson set up The Spectrum Pharmacist in 2020, influenced by two of her children who were diagnosed with autism. She urges families to consider a pharmacist as part of their healthcare team. While autism isn't treated with medication, many of its co-existing conditions can be. Anderson, who still works as a hospital pharmacist, says she was routinely inundated with questions from parents about what medication was best for their child. She says an autistic person might require medication for insomnia and anxiety, for example, while those with ADHD can access medication that targets the primary condition, which can help significantly.

> 'Overall, her diagnosis has been a positive impact on our family. She says, on the medication "my brain feels calm".'

During our research, parents frequently told us of the benefit of medicine for treating symptoms of ADHD, particularly in providing focus for their child. As one parent noted: 'Before my child was medicated, I would introduce myself to parents and they'd ask which child was mine. I'd point him out and their response was, "Oh, yes, everyone knows him!" Sadly, I knew it wasn't for his outstanding behaviour.'

Because medication varies widely, we suggest you seek the support of a doctor and pharmacist to understand the best path for your child. For example, Anderson says some medications are immediate-release (short-acting), while others act over an extended time. Different limits on medications also apply in different states and territories, and problematically, some medications do not have the desired effect on some patients. Medication for anxiety or depression is one example of this. If a child suffers both conditions, which should be addressed first? This is why medical guidance is so important.

Anderson says it's important to remember that at the centre of the diagnosis is a 'beautiful child who sees the world differently' and you don't 'necessarily want them to have to conform to a neurotypical way. At the same time, you want them to have all the opportunities that the neurotypicals have available. There are lots of scenarios where medication is not appropriate, but in some cases, it can be a life changer.'

Anderson, who was Victoria's Pharmacist of the Year in 2022, offers the following advice to parents who are seeking a diagnosis for their child:

- Write notes in the lead-up to your medical appointment. 'If an example of your child's behaviour comes up from a teacher or at home, write down what was happening beforehand, what happened during and what happened after. This will give you a clear idea of whether your child is just having a bad day or not'.

- Plan the list of questions you would like your doctor to answer, before making an informed decision. For example: 'If this medication is used, what can we expect? What sort of doses? What are the adverse effects we should consider?' Given many children have sensory challenges, parents should also ask about the different colours, sizes and textures of the medication available.
- If you start exploring online, as all of us are inclined to do, head for reputable sites: 'Be very careful about where you get your information.'
- A team approach might involve medication and therapy in various mixes, so be open to what might help your child.

Dr Jessica Hill is deputy director of The University of Queensland Animal-Assisted Interventions Alliance. Her interest in autism research is both professional and personal. With four younger autistic siblings, whom she supports, Hill's focus is on animal-assisted therapy, both canine and equine. Her PhD looked at how canine-assisted therapy could help autistic children. She decided to become an OT after her family experienced challenges trying to navigate the education system. On receiving the diagnosis for one of her brothers, the school 'actually told my parents he wasn't welcome there anymore'.

Hill and her mother were 'burnt out from the education system' and none of her siblings finished school. Originally wanting to become a teacher, Hill changed to occupational therapy where she thought she could make more of a difference. She saw how her siblings related to animals, compared to humans, and decided to incorporate that into her private OT sessions with autistic children to help build rapport.

'[My siblings] just wanted to spend a lot of time with the animals and if we went away, they wanted to return to the house to be with the animals.' Two of Hill's siblings live with her now, and she says her own dogs are drawn strongly to them. Seeing the connection with her siblings prompted her own research and training, which she then implemented into her practice.

'It was like night and day, in regard to engaging the kids in my sessions. I can't really explain how different it was.'

She says labrador mixed breeds, such as labradoodles, were very successful. 'My clients are able to communicate with animals non-verbally. Also, the dogs don't place any expectations on the kids.' She provides an example of a simple handwriting exercise, where a child might write a recipe to make a dog cupcake. 'The animals don't care how the writing is done.'

STIGMA, LABELS AND OTHER CHALLENGES

While early diagnosis, medication and therapy can help clear a pathway to success, many find the same pathway covered in weeds. Crucially, a lack of access to a diagnosis can stifle a child's forward journey. The reasons for this are usually geographic or economic, or both. Therapy requires money, so do specialists' assessments. This raises an important equity issue in the diagnosis and treatment of neurodivergencies. Waiting lists to receive a diagnosis can delay opportunities for support, especially in rural and regional areas, where families can sit in a queue for two years, or more. As one mother explained: 'We lived rurally and had to take a day off each week to access speech therapy 300 kilometres away.' Some families lived in towns that had no specialists, or only a single psychologist, who had closed their books to new families. Others had to borrow money – up to $7000 in one case – to relocate to the city and access a diagnosis. Another parent from regional Australia told us: 'If you think you are having a problem in the city, think again. It's a thousand times worse out here, it's the wild, wild west.'

Bonning understands diagnostic challenges, and recognises that delays can have a flow-on effect. Because support services are often not available in regional areas, families are having to get on waiting lists in city areas, which adds to even longer waiting lists.

One mother described the lengthy process to see specialists: 'First an eleven-month wait for a paediatrician and then a further twelve-month wait for a private assessment. I also sent forms off for a public assessment two years ago, as I felt it would be more objective, however I never heard back.' Another told us: 'My daughter was diagnosed at fifteen. She told me she thought she had autism at age thirteen. It took about two years to follow through with the GP, waiting for referrals to the paediatrician, then waiting lists for a psychologist to do the assessment. My daughter became very despondent, upset and lethargic.' Or this: 'My child was diagnosed with Level 2 autism at age seven. We waited two years for the assessment. We are in regional WA and had a different paediatrician more-or-less every appointment. They alternated opinions between autism and ADHD.' And a final example: 'It takes so long to get help. We're four years in … and only just got a proper autism diagnosis last month and no ADHD diganosis yet. The first two years we couldn't get on waitlists; the last two years have been a waste of time and money.'

According to many clinicians, divorce is also more common in families with ND children and this can throw up additional challenges. Different parenting styles and bitter disputes can have a huge impact on an autistic child, particularly around diagnosis and support. As one parent noted: 'She doesn't want to go [to the second parent's house] but is completely disempowered. She assumes a beige demeanour and she just neutralises her environment.' Adjusting to different routines, different boundaries, different foods and different bedtimes can have detrimental impacts on any child, but particularly on ND kids.

The stigma for parents with ADHD children is also cause for concern, which many parents indicated in response to our survey. One mother felt that she was being blamed for her child's behaviour: 'It's just bad parenting or just feral kids or just new-aged hype. Even at nine, [my son] is very aware that some people don't believe him or think he is choosing to be naughty.'

> *'I'm so happy I finally know what's going on with our son and how his brain works. I've been able to have more patience, understanding and compassion for him.'*

Shame often follows a parent out of the diagnosis room: 'The guilt I feel is intense – is it my fault having a child later in life? Is it because me and my husband's genes mismatch?' Another parent said: 'I wish we had been guided to an earlier diagnosis – no one gave us clear confirmation along the way that we should seek further assessments.'

A confirmed diagnosis also brings with it a label; and for parents this can present either a real difficulty – preventing many from seeking a diagnosis in the first place – or a wonderful opportunity to access support and improve their lives. 'I get angry with people who don't want a label,' one mother said. 'It's not about them. It's about their child. Interventions help and they learn how to navigate the world for themselves.'

Author Kate Foster says a label, if delivered positively, can empower a child – 'I'm just me and this is how I do things.' She says many parents are 'terrified of words and they avoid labelling their children because of negative connotations'.

> *'An autism diagnosis isn't as scary as it seems. A proper diagnosis opens the right doors to the supports you need.'*

Kristy Forbes is an autism and neurodiversity support specialist. She formally identifies as autistic, ADHD and has PDA, as well as being a parent to four ND children. Her take is as honest as it is refreshing. 'I spent the first five years trying to cure my child's autism. So, I was one of those parents before I knew better.' She also observes an irony that exists when some parents, who do not want their child to be labelled as autistic, then claim autistic people are too rigid or inflexible. She says that until she was in her thirties, she thought she was 'inherently flawed and broken'. That was until she realised, 'I am exactly who I am supposed to be and was always supposed to be. The things that have been causing me stress and anxiety and trauma were mostly because I was not made for those things. And those things were not made for me.'

What allowed her to change her thinking?

'How in love with my own autistic children I am,' she says. She discovered she was autistic when her children were being assessed. 'If your child doesn't have a label that makes accessing support possible, they will end up with other labels like "lazy", "procrastinator", "school refuser".'

DIAGNOSIS, LABELS AND LANGUAGE

THE IMPORTANCE OF LANGUAGE

The language used in popular media to describe and discuss neurodiversity is front and centre in how it is portrayed to broader society, and this also flows through to families considering a diagnosis. The ND community have adopted neuro-affirming language to avoid the stigma associated with labels that are attached to a diagnosis. What do 'special education', 'special needs' and 'special school' mean, for example? Or even 'mainstream'?

'They're actually quite offensive,' Kate Foster says, as are references to scales or ratings that are often attached to the autism spectrum. 'I've been asked during school visits, how autistic are you out of ten?' she says. 'I find it very strange that we have these scores, and I appreciate it all comes down to funding and support, but autism is now being understood as a colour wheel, rather than a sliding spectrum. All of us have different traits – we just present differently.'

As an example, Asperger Syndrome – the former word for autism Level 1 – is no longer widely used, and yet hundreds of books and academic papers and diagnoses still term it this way.

Numeric levels may no longer be supported by the neuro-affirming community, but the system still requires them to unlock support. The *Diagnostic and Statistical Manual of Mental Disorders, Fifth Edition* (DSM-5) defines three levels of autism. Level 1 signals that a person requires support, while Level 2 denotes substantial support is required. Level 3 indicates a more severe disability, where the person requires very substantial support. While these levels are still used in diagnoses, they are increasingly eschewed by many in the autism community, who prefer the broader autism category, without specific levels.

Forbes says the discussion about low- and high-functioning autistic labels and categories isn't useful. 'For people who are labelled severely autistic, they are completely undermined. And for people who are labelled mildly autistic, they are completely overestimated, or not believed, or gaslit. We are autistic people.'

'I hate the word "diagnosis",' Sutton agrees. 'And I hate the word "label".' Diagnosis medicalises neurodivergence; labels can carry a negative inference. 'I like the word "explanation".' The problem is that the government funding system, or NDIS, means families have to play the game to access support. 'As therapists, we all need to advocate for the NDIS to move away from that very medicalised model,' Sutton says. 'Wouldn't it be exciting if people just got the help they needed, regardless of what their actual diagnosis was. If we moved away from using the term "diagnosis" to using "explanation", then all of a sudden we're shifting the stigma.'

Another word to prompt Sutton's ire, is "refuses", as it relates to school refusal – an outdated term to describe a student's inability to go to school. 'It's not school refusal! It's terrifying. He's not refusing to participate; he's unable to participate,' she says. Sutton suggests using the terms 'non-speaking' over 'nonverbal', 'non-autistic' or 'neurotypical' for what many people call a 'normal person' and 'co-occurring' instead of 'co-morbidity'. Within the autistic community, many advocate for Autism Spectrum Difference or simply autism, over Autism Spectrum Disorder. She also recommends using the term 'individual needs' or 'specific needs' over 'special needs'; and 'situationally mute' rather than 'selectively mute'.

Emily Hammond is autistic and has ADHD. She is also a speech pathologist, illustrator and mother to three ND children. She runs a popular Facebook support group called NeuroWild and says much of the terminology used to describe the ND community has been thrust on them without consent. 'A lot of it is very misplaced because it comes from a neurotypical person's perception of how we live and what our struggles might be. So, at the moment, there is a strong consensus for the kind of language that we like. We're just autistic,' she says.

QUICK TIPS FOR DIAGNOSIS

Dr Bronwyn Sutton provides the following advice for parents and carers who are considering seeking a ND diagnosis:

- Trust your gut instinct at all times.
- Be open to hearing feedback from your child's educators – your child may act differently in different social settings.
- Embrace neurodiversity: a diagnosis is an explanation of your child's challenges. Understanding your ND child will help you explain their uniqueness and struggles to teachers and relatives.
- Find two wise therapists who will support you, as well as your child. Rather than just observing the therapists at work, practise what to do, and learn from them.
- Consider rating your therapist not only on how they work with your child, but on how well they educate the adults around your child. This will ultimately help change your child's environment so that they don't need to struggle.
- Connect with other parents and autistic adults.
- Choose sources of information carefully – start with Australian Government or university websites, or your state-based autism organisations.

PART I: FRIENDSHIPS

2. FRIENDSHIPS IN PRIMARY SCHOOL

Until a child is six or even eight years old, the differences they see between themselves and other kids are obvious, particularly when it comes to race and gender. Apart from that, children think they are all cast from the same mould. But, at around Year 1, children start to discern how others have personalities or abilities different from their own, and that's when they start asking questions and see themselves as not 'fitting in'. Many of the neurodivergent (ND) children who responded to our survey confirmed this: 'I don't understand why I feel the way I feel. It feels strange, and sometimes out of my control'; 'I would love to have friends who accept me for who I am, and don't think I'm weird or hate me.'

> *'Why do I have to be less me and more everyone else. Don't I matter as me?'*

Feeling left out or sidelined by their peers has negative impacts on children's self-esteem, confidence and enjoyment of life. There's no doubt that ND children are feeling isolated, lonely, bullied and misunderstood. Friendship is a game-changer for all children, and the role of parents here should not be underestimated.

In more cases than not, ND kids are aware of their differences, but this is not being understood by their neurotypical (NT) peer groups. As one ND kid observed: 'My biggest challenge is that everything feels hard for me that the other kids just do so easy. Making friends is okay, but I am never their favourite and they get sick of me, and I don't always understand the jokes they make … so it feels like they are making fun of me and I hate that. Sometimes I pretend to understand, but they know and think I am dumb. I have gotten into a few fights this year because I get angry really quickly, but even when I try to walk away, they think it is funny to follow me and tease me. [Then] I get in trouble because they tell the teachers a different story – I get confused and muddled, and they think I am lying. I would just like to have a couple of friends that understand me and don't think I am a weirdo.'

> **'Making friends is easy. Keeping them is hard.'**

As our research revealed, this also poses challenges for parents and carers. 'I love my children to the end of the world, I love them for them, and at times their ND thinking impresses me, but there is also grief and distress at how hard life is for them in a NT world.'

Parents are often grappling with how to manage a child's social life without impacting their self-esteem: 'This year has been the first year (he is in Year 3) that he has felt different from his peers. Another girl called him stupid and weird, the word "weird" stuck with him more. He was really down for weeks, resigned and saying, "I guess I am weird".'

FITTING IN

Play dates are at the heart of the primary-school experience. Birthday parties, especially, are a colourful way to celebrate a milestone, surrounded by friends, filling smartphone albums with photographs of a child taking centrestage, relishing in relaxed rules around eating cake, being feted by siblings and friends, and smiling gleefully before candles are extinguished to badly sung lyrics of *Happy Birthday*. Part of the fun is in the planning. The invitation that outlines the rules: when, where and what time? Should there be a theme? And the closing date for RSVPs, so we know who will walk through the door with a smile, and even a gift. As that RSVP date closes in, children will inquire who is coming to their birthday party. Is Will coming? What about Arjun? Amelia? Cho? Who else is coming?

But for many children birthday parties are the cause of heartbreak; a reminder that they have no friends, and of how often difference is shunned. It's also a reminder that friendships can be excruciatingly hard and the influence of some parents can be downright disheartening.

All children miss out on birthday party invites at some point, but what if you miss out every time? What if you're never invited? For ND primary school-aged children, particularly, this can be their story. As one parent told us: 'He doesn't get invited to any birthday parties. Breaks my heart. He's not mean, just misunderstood. He misses all the social intelligence.'

> **'No RSVPs from kids to his birthday party and no invitation to others either.'**

Other parents relayed similar experiences for their kids: 'Never been invited to one party, and one year was the only child out of the whole class to be excluded from a birthday party'; 'He has no friends. Not invited to a birthday party since Year 2. Unable to make peer friends.'

These answers pull the cover off myriad issues circling early friendships for children who think differently to their peers. Both boys and girls are subject to this treatment, which raises questions about how we, as a society, view diversity. In our survey, ND parents believed that exclusive behaviours often stem from a NT parent, who encourages their child not to befriend a peer they consider 'odd' or 'quirky' or 'hard work'. An irony stands out here, too, when the attributes of autistic children are frequently observed as being funny and loyal, open and honest, with a strong sense of social justice. It only further underscores the value of ND kids learning how to read themselves and others, understanding the process of making and keeping friends, and teaching all children the value of what difference can offer.

> *'They seem to like me, but I don't understand why they don't invite me places. They say their parents say I can't come over.'*

Parents of ND children become experts at changing the narrative around missed occasions to ease the hurt for their child: 'This is better because we can go to the zoo and you can buy something from the gift shop.' Or, 'We'll have dinner with the whole family including your cousins!' But as young as five, children can see they are being excluded at a milestone celebration. They turn up to school and hear other kids excitedly talk about Jack's party on the weekend. That sense of not belonging, of being shut out or ostracised, only increases as children climb through primary school and become teenagers.

STUMBLING BLOCKS

So, what are the most difficult friendship issues that trip up children who are different from their peers? How can they navigate the playground where bullying, teasing, humiliation and rejection can become a hierarchical currency? The characteristics of neurodivergence that often create social stumbling blocks are the same ones that can single them out in class and can impact young adults in relationships and even in the workplace. Of course, these traits are part of the personality of many children but can be more pronounced and recur more often for ND kids. In addition, autistic children can be between two and four years behind their peers, developmentally, when it comes to friendship.

> **LACK OF IMPULSE CONTROL:** 'My daughter has only a few friends and can be very blunt. One of her friends was playing with another friend which really upset my daughter, so she sent her a message to say she hates her. We had a conversation about friendships and behaviour, and after apologising [she] was able to keep the friendship, but I am concerned this will not always be the case.'
>
> **BLACK-AND-WHITE THINKING:** 'When my son was eight, a PE teacher instructed the kids to have a two-second drink at the tap before continuing on. When the boy in front of my son took twenty seconds to have a drink, my son shoved him in the back and told him off. He takes everything literally and thought the PE teacher genuinely wanted the kids to only drink for two seconds.'
>
> **WANTING TO BE 'BOSS':** 'She wants to be in charge and control everything and when it doesn't go her way, lashes out and

can be quite hurtful/nasty, thus pushing friends away and making herself a target to be excluded.' And: 'He finds the "unpredictability" of play with peers difficult, therefore has always preferred to play with younger children where he is in control.' Or: 'My nine-year-old son struggled at school with lunchtime friendships because unless he was choosing the game and in charge, he wasn't interested. He wouldn't play with anyone unless he was making the rules and controlling the experience.'

NOT READING SOCIAL CUES: 'He is very literal and often misses social cues. He will do or say things that aren't appropriate with no realisation.' And: 'She has no capacity for empathy or seeing someone else's perspective.'

NOT UNDERSTANDING THE TENETS OF A FRIENDSHIP, BEYOND THE IMMEDIATE: 'He is friends with everyone but has no one close to him. So, he tends to give kids an ultimatum, like: "If you don't meet me in the library when it's open, I'll poke you with my pencil." He doesn't realise that it's not acceptable and that [his behaviour] has an adverse effect on kids.'

A STRONG SENSE OF SOCIAL JUSTICE: 'Sometimes children can get sick of his black-and-white thinking at playtime – for instance, if someone cheats or does the wrong thing, he can get very upset and fixate on this.'

NOT UNDERSTANDING SARCASM AND BEING GULLIBLE: 'My son was at after-school care and came across two older boys who were making a tall tower out of some huge blocks. My son asked, "Can I push that over?" When the older boys said, "Yeah sure" in a sarcastic tone, my son didn't get the sarcasm. All he heard was "Yes". So, he pushed the tower over and the older boys called him a moron. I found my son weeping in the corner of the playground at pick-up time.'

REPORTING MINOR MISDEMEANOURS: 'My autistic child takes rules very seriously and will often dob on classmates who are breaking the rules. When I try and point out that this isn't their job, they look at me baffled. Rules, in their head, must always be followed.'

Tony Attwood says, while peers can be compassionate and caring, when it comes to status within the group, allegiance to an autistic person isn't always valued and they are not seen as 'cool'. He recently had a client who told him that on finishing high school, one peer told her that it 'just wasn't cool to be seen' with her. And what did Attwood tell his client? That her friend would 'eventually grow up and appreciate who you really are' – honest, reliable, determined – skills her peer group might have been too immature to appreciate.

'His words: "I never know if someone is actually my friend."'

Often, when primary school-aged children are excluded from groups at lunchtime, or know others are invited to places they are not, Attwood will take out a big piece of paper and ask them to nominate their qualities. He asks their parents, too. Perhaps being kind will come up. An ability to spot errors. Being social-justice oriented. Attwood says it's important to see the advantage of attributes over a lifespan. This isn't a lesson for ND children, but for all children; 'Your peer group doesn't appreciate them yet.'

He tells another story: this time it's a young man he began seeing fifteen years ago, when the boy was three. 'And he says,

"I'm useless. I'm hopeless, I'll never be a success." I said, "Wait a minute, when I first met you at three, you weren't toilet trained and you weren't talking. Now, your mum has a terminal illness, and you're her caregiver." Good God, those are the most beautiful personality qualities you could ever wish for.'

In our survey, children regularly asked their parents to help 'fix' friendships at school. And there is no doubt that teaching autistic children and others the tenets of being a good friend starts at home. Firstly, Attwood urges parents to give positive feedback when a child shows a friendship skill, such as caring or sharing. 'Please compliment them for doing that, because for many autistic kids, the only feedback they get is when they do something wrong and have to be corrected.' Secondly, certain friendship ingredients needed to be taught specifically. 'In autism, you need to explain the logic that you might not have to explain to others,' he says.

> *'Other kids say things I don't understand but I'm learning it's sometimes called sarcasm, or it's "just a saying".'*

For Dr Wesley Turner, friendship comes down to the idea of synchrony. 'What friendship is, in my mind at least, is the continual refinement and revision of an interpersonal interaction with someone who mirrors us to some degree – we have more similarities than differences'. We feel a connection or an attunement. We know how they are feeling most of the time. But a 'double empathy problem' can arise. This is a theory that says when people of very different experiences interact, they can find it difficult to empathise with each other and find common ground. Autistic children, or those with

ADHD, might find it difficult to understand a NT child – and vice versa. 'If you are from Fiji, you will understand that way of life, perhaps better than how the Spanish live,' Turner explains. His advice is to find similarities. Sometimes this is referred to as 'finding your tribe'. But Turner admits that this can also be confusing for some children, who will respond by saying, 'But I don't know who my tribe is, and I don't know where to find them.' His advice is to steer ND kids towards team sports or other interests or activities so they can experience situations and environments where they can see similarities and not feel different – and where NT children will also see the similarities.

Turner provides another avenue for children to open their minds to friendships. Often, we teach kids to look outside of themselves to other people, and ND children can find that hard. He suggests 'mentalising', or encouraging the child to see how they are feeling in any particular moment. For example, by asking specific questions: 'What do I notice in my body? Am I tired? Am I having pleasure? Displeasure? Am I alert? Am I low? Am I thirsty? Am I hungry?' To know what someone else is thinking or feeling, a child (or adult) needs to 'check in' with themselves first – it's a two-way street. 'If we don't have a good radar for our internal experiences, we actually can't tell what someone else is thinking or feeling.'

How do you teach a five-year-old autistic child, for example, how to understand their own feelings? Turner answers our question with his own. 'How does a child learn when they're injured?' We've all seen a child trip, see a spot of blood, and then look to a parent. 'Should I be hurt? Should I be crying?' Turner says an autistic child might not make eye contact but will orient in the same way. 'They will still have this pause moment where they're not entirely sure. They haven't got that bank [of knowledge] yet of determining what to do. That's when we want to be – as parents, as friends and support people – helping them by providing options and guides,' he says. We shouldn't tell them what they're feeling, but 'if we don't give them anything, we can't expect them to know. They need to learn,' he says.

Kate Foster is an autistic author whose first book, *Paws*, was published in 2021. Aimed at children aged seven to twelve, it tells the story of primary schooler Alex and his dog, Kevin, at Australia's best dog show. Eleven-year-old Alex is autistic, and is frightened of going to high school, which is just a few months away. Alex realises he needs to get some friends by his side, and he sets out to create a 'three-step, foolproof, friend-making plan'. But like all good plots, it doesn't go the way it should, and Alex finds making friends much harder than he expected.

Foster says she writes to escape and has been doing it since she could hold a pen: 'It's a great way to process the world as well'. Growing up, Foster didn't realise she was autistic. 'I knew I was different, so I think writing was a way of making sense of everything and giving myself an outlet.' She wants to make it easier for the next generation of children, including her own son, to see the value of connection and for all children to see 'what they have in common with kids who might be different to them'.

THE ROLE PARENTS PLAY IN FRIENDSHIPS

For the parents of those children excluded from peer groups, it's a difficult path. The saying that 'you're only as happy as your least happy child' has been attributed to numerous sources, including the Bible. But watching your child being rejected over and over again can also impact parents. As one parent told us: 'He has spent most of his lunches recently on his own and has said, "I have no one to hang out with me, so sometimes I just go to the office and pretend to be sick so I can stay in sick bay".' Another told us: 'He received his first birthday invitation from a friend in Year 5. I cried. He thought he had friends but was never truly included. When we asked what he did at lunch, he would tell us he watched as his friends played.'

The involvement of NT parents was also perceived as having negative impacts on all children: 'We have been told not to see my neighbours anymore as [my daughter] had two meltdowns at their last birthday party in May and I had to remove her ... I was sent a message to say, "we are done".'

The parents of ND children can be angry or heartbroken at the treatment meted out by others, while the parents of NT children who don't embrace difference may have undue influence over their own children's behaviour, even encouraging them to steer clear of those who are not mirror images of their clan. As one mother said: 'Friendship challenges are more from the parents. They won't allow children over and make up reasons for why they can't catch up outside of school. They have other kids over.'

This is not on our children, this is on us, surely? After all, if it takes a village to raise a child, it takes a village to understand the differences that exist among our children. Attwood agrees. The guest list is drawn up, usually, by the child. 'I think it would be good for the parents of the other children to have some degree of responsibility,' he reminds us. For autistic children, he says an invitation to one party, from one friend, might make all the difference. 'When I look at the long-term success rate, it's often having one friend, not forever, not for all the school years, but at least you've proved that you've done it. So just having one friend, one birthday invitation, can mean "I can do it."'

This view is widely supported by other experts. Turner says 'difference' can scare many people, including adults. 'What happens from a neurological point of view, is that when we perceive uncertainty and we don't know what to do, we perceive it, more often than not, as a threat.' That means people might avoid confronting an issue. 'So, you unfortunately see a lot of people just saying things like, "Well, let's not invite Timmy around. You know, he's a lovely child, but ..."'

> 'It broke my heart to see his loneliness when he realised he had been rejected, again and again.'

Of course there are exceptions, and the impact of that can bring joy both to a child and their parents. This is from one parent: 'My son's friend had a birthday party and his mum contacted me to ask if there was anything she could do to make sure he had a great time. She had all the details ready for me and had options if it got too much. It meant so much that they wanted him to be there, and they wanted him to enjoy himself.'

ADHD coach Tamara Rosier understands the heartbreak parents feel when their child is excluded. Her advice is for the adults to separate their emotions from those of their child and focus on one-on-one time with them instead. She says those with ADHD can run three years behind their peers in terms of peer-to-peer relationships, and parents can help their child gain valuable experiences. Rosier says that time would prove much more fruitful than missed birthday parties. 'Go fishing. Do all the things with the kid in one-on-one time because you're teaching them how to be together. Lock away your phone. Ask questions. Don't try and lecture your child when you're rollerblading. Just ask questions and focus on those activities.'

But what do you say to your eight- or ten-year-old who has been excluded?

'It is hard to watch your child be disappointed and left out,' Rosier says. But parents need to be a rock for their child and ask themselves, 'How can I help this child express his or her emotions, but not wallow in them?'

Talk about it, and assure them it is okay to be sad, and then ask – depending on their age – what do they want to do 'to get the sadness out of their body'?

They might want to cry or take a bat to a tree. 'Do they want to jump on a trampoline?' When Rosier asked one young boy, he told her he wanted to cuddle his mum and watch a home-decorating channel. For older children, Rosier says parents need to 'manage themselves'. 'If the parents are like, "Oh well, I never liked [the friend] anyway, she's a nasty girl" – what will their child take from this?' Rosier encourages parents to remain neutral. You need to say, 'I'm really sorry, that hurts. How do you want to manage this?' She also suggests parents consider the three values they want their child to learn, and use friendship spikes as a means of teaching those. Try and use incidents of rejection to teach resilience, where a child learns to bounce back; or kindness, where it is important to ensure parents don't 'talk trash' about other children.

Certainly, the parents of primary school-aged children reported a heart-rending level of bullying of ND children. Young students arrived home with bruises but explained, 'the other kids didn't mean it'. We heard of some who had received revolting messages on Messenger Kids. One child reported being flicked in the neck repeatedly, while the teacher's back was turned, and until they retaliated. As one mother said: 'Middle school! Freaking brutal. Other kids were awfully cruel and just intolerant of difference.' Sadly, this story was not isolated.

Our survey revealed that ND kids have had their lunches stolen, eaten and tramped on, they are regularly teased or excluded from games, or told to disappear. There were reports of primary school kids being tricked into spreading porn or signing up to adult dating sites. The stories are more graphic and more serious in high school, which is discussed in the next chapter. But it begins after difference is recognised by peers, usually in primary and middle school. As one parent said: 'There are no words to describe what we have been through trying to mainstream our kids.'

MEAN GIRLS

Examples of girls being mean to each other were widespread: 'She managed to make one friend this year, finally,' one mother said. 'That girl wasn't nice and the friendship has ended. [Now] my daughter can't be friends with others in the group because the main girl she was friends with will get mad.' And this, from another mother: 'She's ten [with autism] – two girls came to her party on Sunday as part of a group of six. [On] Tuesday they wrote a note saying they wouldn't be her friend anymore. She felt completely betrayed. The girls couldn't justify why they did it. They had no direct reason. Trying to explain girl bitchiness as some sort of developmental phase to a ND girl is hard.'

Parents report girls' treatment of ND peers can often be 'bistrategic', a term clinical psychologist Dr Mary Kaspar, author of *The Popular Girls*, defines as a combination of being both nice and mean – think of the characters in *Mean Girls* or *Gossip Girl*. Often, the bullying culprits – both boys and girls – faced no consequences. In the words of one parent: 'Girls are not able to see my daughter for who she is. She's left out, shut out and not invited to hang out at lunch or parties and play dates.' Another parent said: 'Girls can be so hard. Their advanced language skills can be used to target, isolate and bully ND girls.'

> **'Girls are mean to ND kids [who] don't know how to "play the emotional game".'**

'The kids who can communicate and come up with a story win. If your communication is lacking, you pretty much have no chance. They twist things around. They manipulate that situation,' one mother said. 'Teachers always believe the NT kids' versions of events over the ND kids',' said another.

So, why are ND children so susceptible or vulnerable to bullying?

'They're vulnerable because they don't react in the same way,' Turner says. 'And in some instances, unfortunately, people get joy out of seeing someone not know how to cope with something. That is bullying. When you have someone who's so different – because their neurology is different, how they process information is different, also what they expect or predict is different – it means that they're always going to be open to being vulnerable.'

Within society, this is what we see mirrored in the treatment of different races and cultures and sexualities. If a ten-year-old was sitting across from Turner, explaining a bullying incident, he'd respond by 'validating the hell out of their pain'. Don't dismiss it or skip over how hurtful it might be. Children need to understand what's going on. 'I would help them connect with their internal experience to understand what they're feeling.' That would help them decipher what is right and wrong for them. 'Do they have power in a school environment to defend themselves? It depends. In a lot of cases, no, which is absolutely horrible, but it's really important for them to know that it is wrong'.

> *'Girls are very hard to understand. My daughter doesn't pick up on social nuances and can be easily mocked without her knowing. She has lost friends because their parents don't like the way she behaves.'*

Clubs, driven by interest, and team activities can both offer a buffer against bullying and help build positive friendship experiences. Turner says, 'If we have a shared environment, it's like, "Hey, we're all playing football together right now." And it makes things a hell of a lot easier.'

Turner endorses drama classes as a way of building interpersonal skills: 'I recommend it very strongly – anything that is performative'. But with a caveat: children must also continue to focus on what they are feeling internally, so they don't perfect the art of masking their condition.

PRIMARY SCHOOL FRIENDSHIP TIPS

1. Explicitly teach your child what a good friendship looks like, and feels like, as well as the small acts or behaviours that can strengthen friendships. Examples include giving your full attention, nodding when your friend is sharing a story or information, and following up on things your friend is concerned about. If they mention their grandma is unwell or their dog is at the vet, you remember this information and the following day check in with your friend.
2. Join clubs – drama, chess, robotics, sports and debating are often offered within school lunch breaks. Choose something that will align with your child's interests, so their knowledge and input will be valued by the group.
3. Focus on your child having friends outside of the school bubble. Look at groups and organisations outside of school hours that your child might be interested and engaged in.
4. As an NT parent, ask the teacher: 'Which kids in the class aren't getting invited to play dates or parties?' Invite these kids on play dates and to your child's next party. This may be the only invitation that ND child receives this year.
5. Model acceptance and inclusion at home. Pay attention to how your child speaks about other kids. If you hear your child making fun of ND (or any other) kids, chat to them privately about it. Remind them of the importance of kindness, talk about the value in difference and diversity, think of times when they have been left out and how good it feels to be included, and watch movies like *Wonder*.

3. FRIENDSHIPS IN HIGH SCHOOL

OVER THE CHRISTMAS HOLIDAYS, CHRISTINE'S son spent long days fishing, swimming, riding bikes and building forts with friends who lived in the local neighbourhood. The boys shared sleepovers, and Christine's son generously used his own pocket money to buy bait and hot chips for his friends. 'Unfortunately, two days into high school, my son had been excluded. With more kids around, my son had more difficulty reading the social cues and fitting in. The group that had been accepting of him over the holidays no longer wanted to spend time with him,' she told us. Alice's daughter had the opposite problem. While her peers spent the holidays shopping, going to the movies and having sleepovers, she sat in her room. Alice realises she only made it worse by constantly asking why her daughter wasn't with friends. Those stories are mirrored time and again, as neurodivergent (ND) children transfer from primary school into high school. Elijah is thirteen and his mother has a stack of stories. In one incident, two peers stood either side of her son and hit their heads with their hands, saying over and over, 'I'm autistic'. 'It breaks my heart. There's not a lot I can do. Sometimes they leave him alone and sometimes they don't.'

High school can be tricky for many children, but particularly ND students. Most ND children, like most neurotypical (NT) children, are kind and want to be friends with everybody. But the new school landscape throws up significant challenges. Some children are still naive; others are more worldly, with hundreds of friends on social media. Cliques develop quickly. Bonding can abruptly turn to bullying. Boys often find 'roasting' each other brings kudos, even when the jokes are homophobic, sexist or racist. Behaviour that was accepted in primary school is suddenly viewed as 'weird'.

'In high school she stood still whilst all her primary school friends moved on. She was isolated and a target for bullies.'

As our research revealed, ND kids can then inadvertently become targets. As one mother told us: 'I got a phone call from the school saying my son had jumped out a window – his friends were playing superheroes, and he was Spider-Man, and was dared to do it.' In some cases, often after being baited, ND teens can also become the instigators.

The stories told to us around high-school friendships spanned more than torment though; they showed how belonging is paramount, and there were often negative consequences for teenagers who were trying their hardest to 'fit in'. In the words of one parent: 'My daughter was going to have some school friends over, she was so excited. She said the girls ignored her at school, so she cancelled it. I think she just missed some social cues. My beautiful girl was *soooo* upset.'

Responses to our survey from the parents of teenagers revealed how friendship struggles played out in a multitude of ways:

- 'His difficulty is with maintaining close relationships. He would interact with different people each day, depending on what he was currently interested in or doing.'
- 'My daughter thinks of friends, other than her best friend, as friends of the best friend [but not of hers] – she essentially ignores them and interacts only with the best friend.'
- 'At school he eats lunch with a few kids, but it is more a five-minute chat about games and the rest sitting playing computer games next to each other.'
- 'As she's hit the tweens she has struggled to adapt to the different "play" the other girls do now. She still wants to run and play actively, whereas most girls her age just want to talk. She also takes things literally and misses social cues.'
- 'She processes things in a very black-and-white way. It's either right or wrong. Maintaining relationships with her peers is so difficult because they don't have the patience to deal with how she takes things. It's not always her fault, but she also finds it very difficult to accept situations and forgive.'
- 'He can struggle to read the room. He also gets "peopled out" pretty quickly and can shut down.'
- 'My daughter has struggled with friends her whole school career [currently in Year 9]. We have tried everything. Unless you have a ND child, I don't think you can understand what it's like.'
- 'She panics and can respond impulsively. She's so soft but she always lashes out, and then wonders why the few friends she has don't forgive [her] immediately.'

WHY FRIENDSHIP MATTERS

Clinical psychologist and author Dr Mary Kaspar says friendship really matters to all children. She points to the future-proofing research conducted by the Black Dog Institute, which in 2019 launched a long-term study into adolescent mental health. A total of 6388 high-school students from 134 Australian schools completed annual questionnaires. The study was commenced when those students were in Year 8, with a mean age of 13.9 years, and was followed up annually over a period of five years. Results indicated concerning levels of peer connectedness in the general high-school population, with one-quarter not making friends easily, almost one-third feeling like they don't 'belong' at school, and almost one in five feeling 'lonely' at school. The results were similar in metropolitan and regional areas, and sightly higher for males than females.

> *'He has no real-life friends and can only interact online.'*

'We know that having supportive, trusting relationships is integral to adolescent teen heath,' Kaspar says. Rates of loneliness were about twice as high in marginalised and minority student groups, including those who had a learning difficulty or a disability. 'That means those social connections are absolutely crucial for reducing loneliness with knock-on effects for mental health and wellbeing.'

Emily Hammond, the brains behind NeuroWild, says one of her most popular downloaded resources is the 'double empathy problem'. She explains it using illustrations of a chat between a beaver and a squirrel. Beavers can make friends and communicate with other beavers, and squirrels with squirrels.

But when beavers and squirrels get together, there can be communication problems. 'It just means that more curiosity and open-mindedness is required, and a whole lot less judgement,' she says. 'We're speaking different languages, essentially, and all of the work is not ours to do alone.'

In Tony Attwood's and Michelle Garnett's clinical experience, they also see some autistic adolescents gravitating towards marginalised teenage groups who 'engage in activities and interests that tend to cause concern for parents'. This might mean they are drawn to drug and alcohol abuse or sex and eating disorders, for example. 'The friendship family "adopts" the autistic teenager, who acquires a new intense interest and may accumulate knowledge from the Internet that the group values.'

Attwood says that while autism delivers wonderful personal traits, one of the 'unfortunate components' can be a sense of pessimism, where the teen looks at their own faults. 'They tend to be incredibly self-critical. And they have a level of expectation greater than their parents, greater than their teachers. And they disappoint themselves. They're not very good at saying, "Nice one, me, I did a good job there". It's, "No, I wasn't good enough".' He says working to change that pessimism and negativity is important. 'Not to be Pollyanna optimistic, but to be more realistic because they often disappoint themselves.'

TEENS, TECH AND SOCIAL MEDIA

Increasingly, ND children are the target of bullying or predatory behaviour on their smart devices. In Tom's case, he sent a full-body naked photo of himself to a stranger online. 'Everything we taught him went out the window,' his mother says. 'He sent photos of himself to someone he thought was his age.' Tom clearly circumvented parental controls to join Instagram; his mother was alerted to it one Saturday morning when he became distraught. 'I've been talking to this girl,' he told her. 'She asked me for some photos and she sent me some, too.' He thought his new friend was thirteen; police later tracked the perpetrator to Nigeria and told his mother they were now routinely receiving between thirty and fifty similar reports a week. This scammer, posing as a teen girl, had demanded Tom send $1500 or 'she' would upload his photos for everyone to see.

'She made him feel special and had been grooming him for a month. I think, with autism, he is more vulnerable because he is so trusting,' his mother told us. 'He didn't question the motive behind any of it.' This is sextortion, which is reaching epidemic proportions in Australia – with boys a growing target.

> *'Her psychologist has deemed her an "at risk" child for child grooming. I'm doing everything I can to prepare her for the outside world.'*

Sarah was a similar age when a group of girls at school bullied her into chatting to strangers via online dating sites. If she refused, they told her they would spread vicious rumours about her. 'And she went down the rabbit hole,' her mother says. Tasting victory, her tormentors also sent her links to more than fifty pornographic websites, before deleting their messages. Parental controls on her smart devices didn't alert Sarah's parents; it was a new level of secrecy she was displaying that prompted concern. And that's when her family discovered that at the age of eleven,

Sarah had joined an adult dating website and was chatting with adult men.

It didn't stop there. Her parents then found pornographic images in her room. 'She gets rejected every day [at school], [but] online there are people who will play around with her and give her what she craves,' her mother says. 'I absolutely don't think it's over. I'm waiting for the next time it happens.'

Tom's and Sarah's experiences are not isolated incidents. Indeed, the vulnerability of ND tweens and teens, who value trust and want to be accepted and fit in, stands out as an opportunity for bullies both offline and online. As one parent observed: 'Her "friends" walk all over her – [they] get hold of her phone and message other people or remove her from group chats.'

The bullying targeting ND children can be relentless. Social media is simply the delivery mode in many cases. All too often, the incidence of online harassment ramps up as children graduate from primary school and head to high school. This transition, with different classrooms, teachers and subjects, is confusing enough, but school also provides an automatic groupthink; a contagion that can deliver persistent and targeted bullying.

As one mother observed: 'I know that as soon as he gets a smart phone, things will change for the worse. This is basically like putting the pokies in his pocket – so much cheap dopamine. I'm worried about where that will lead. It's already a challenge with his school laptop and phone.' She says she is sick of experts saying parents and carers need to teach kids how to have a healthy relationship with technology. 'It's rubbish. Why would we put a highly addictive piece of technology into the hands of a kid who is prone to addictive behaviour and then expect them to self-moderate? It's terrible advice.'

Attwood says he routinely sees in his clinic the traumatic consequences of 'bullying, teasing, humiliation and rejection'. 'Yes, you want them to engage – but who with? And the risk is that it will be an aversive experience [where] the person feels "What's the point, they're always going to be cruel to me".' He says he looks at the profound psychological effects of bullying as a precursor to depression and self-harm. 'One of the major reasons for camouflaging and eating disorders is bullying and teasing, because the person camouflages to fit in so they're not targeted,' he says. The issue here isn't autism; 'It's the attitude of the peer group towards the person,' he says. Attwood is always measured; always calm. But you can hear the frustration in his voice. And this concern is matched by the parents of autistic teenagers.

Even when a child is not being bullied, it doesn't mean they are able to make and keep friends. Of course, some do, they find people who think like them. Or they find friends who share the same interests and a bond builds. Or they find someone, just one friend, who has their back and builds them up. But for many who are seen as different, friendship is a daily struggle, and bullying is commonplace.

Attwood says for autistic teens, a friend is 'more likely to be described as someone with a similar interest'. They might like and talk about the same things but are less likely to swap secrets or show deep affection to each other. They are also more likely to enjoy the same interests they had in their early primary school years, such as Lego and My Little Pony.

This sentiment from one mother is echoed from families nationwide: 'If I had my time again, I would go to a school as low-tech as possible; not one that gives them access to Internet at nine. I'd like schools to take more responsibility than they do now around Internet usage. She needs the control and supervision of a six- or seven-year-old.'

While neurodivergencies bring specific challenges, the role of social media in our schools – primary and secondary – is difficult to chronicle: the disease of comparison it encourages; the access to pornography and groups that can encourage harming behaviours; the entree into grooming and sexual assaults; an obsession with its use, 24/7; the instant gratification it delivers.

The concerns are never-ending, for parents of all children. 'It's not easily fixed in any school,' says one school principal. Another says: 'It's about parent education here, not kids.' And this: 'It's an ongoing challenge.' The head of a school with a high number of autistic students says it was made more difficult with children struggling to read 'social cues or inference or innuendo or sarcasm. They are so easily sucked into inappropriate conversations and it's very, very difficult.'

Psychologist Wesley Turner says teens can get stuck in very unhelpful situations in the search for acceptance. While falling short of a magic bullet, the answer is constant open conversation and dialogue with ND kids. 'It's hard,' he says, before giving an example:

PARENT: What people say isn't always true.

CHILD: Why would people lie?

PARENT: Great question. I don't know, honey. Why do people do a lot of different things? The thing is, that they do, and so we need to work out how to tell when someone's lying or not.

CHILD: What do I do when I can't tell if they're lying or not?

The parent might then focus on the importance of not making immediate decisions and regulating an impulse to respond immediately. Some experts suggest providing our children with ready-made phrases or a script to deal with difficult situations.

Appropriate peer role models, or older role models, such as a guidance counsellor or a trusted teacher, are also important. Ideally, ND kids need 'someone who can speak to them and not in that authoritative parenting way, but more a back-and-forth interaction'. Turner also has this valuable reminder: 'I don't think this is necessarily just an autism or ADHD thing. I think a lot of kids would benefit from this.' Social media is part of our teens' lives. 'It's when do you use it? How do you use it? What's the function of using social media? Are you avoiding connecting with family and people around you? Or is it that you want to see more people who are like you, and have shared interests or experiences?'

TEEN CRUSHES, CURIOSITY AND THE DATING DANCE

Before we take a deep dive into how parents and carers can best help navigate teen friendships, there is one more issue that concerns high-school students that needs attention: romantic relationships. While it's normal as a tween and teen to be interested in sex, and to be attracted to someone else, engaging in more intimate personal relationships can be different for ND kids. With a propensity for black-and-white thinking and miscommunication a common challenge – what is being said might be different from what is heard. Let's take this example, which unfolded in one high school between two ND teens. A fifteen-year-old girl told a male peer that she was interested in him; she wanted to start dating. He pondered the idea and told her he wanted to 'go out' with her too, but he wanted to take it slowly and not make it public to their classmates immediately. One educator explains: 'She interpreted that as though he was ashamed of her. So, she told another boy that she was attracted to him, and they started "dating"'. The first boy was heartbroken. He didn't understand what he had done wrong. 'He is going, "hang on, I just want to get to know you first".'

In another case, a 'break-up' followed a short attachment. But the girl, in this case, refused to accept it, and began stalking her former boyfriend. She wouldn't leave him alone, which created myriad problems. It's customary that adolescence delivers these challenges for almost all teens – it's part of growing up. But with ND teens, there can be added layers of complexity.

Turner says 'masking or camouflaging' can influence attachments, particularly with girls. 'We'll see people saying "yes" to dating when they don't want to. This is something I've seen quite a lot.' He revisits the importance of all teens knowing themselves, and what they are feeling inside. 'I know it's almost like a broken record, but it's really coming back to: What are you feeling? What are you noticing?' Problems, like becoming fixated or overwhelmed, can result from not exploring those internal feelings. Turner believes that a teen who has been dumped by their girlfriend needs their feelings validated. He will first acknowledge how tough it is for them. 'Let's talk about that, and process it and make space for it, to help them get through it. More often than not, the challenge for people who are autistic or have ADHD, or people with attachment trauma, is they haven't had the opportunity to learn how to recognise, organise and respond to their own internal experiences. And that's going to leave them incredibly confused.'

His advice doesn't start and stop with ND teens; surely, all teens need to learn that dating can be a bit like a dance. 'It's learning what dance you like. Do you want to tango? Do you want to do ballet? Do you want to do a little bit of hip-hop?'

Planet Puberty was created as a resource by Family Planning Australia (FPA) in 2021, to help parents educate children with disabilities. Ee-Lin Chang, manager of health promotion at FPA, says the digital resource is about being clear and presenting relevant information that works best for the child. The conversation could be led by either, she says, but it is also important to prepare children for the physical changes they will undergo. 'It's never too early to prepare your child for puberty,' she says, giving the example of hygiene. Or using everyday events, like sharing, to talk about consent.

Cath Hakanson is a sex educator who runs Sex Ed Rescue, an Australian website brimming with tools to help explain sex and puberty. She says education should begin as early as a child is ready. She says parents are often reluctant to talk to their kids about puberty and sex because they fear their child will walk through the school gates and repeat it all. 'That's one of the things that stops them,' she says. 'I think the other thing is that – even if we look at parents who don't have neurodivergent kids – they bloody struggle as well.' Add autism to the mix, and it simply makes it harder.

Hakanson says, 'I'm a big believer in being open and honest. It's very much about using straightforward language, so you need to talk in a way that can't be misinterpreted. So, if they ask you how a motor in a car runs, you would explain it to them in a way that makes sense to them.' She encourages parents to use a simple explanation for a young child; a more detailed explanation for an older child. Conversations about sex require a similar approach. 'If they come home from school and they say, "Mum, what's sex?" You might say, "That's a really good question. Why are you asking?"'

Hakanson says this allows parents to understand the context of the question and what prompted it. For example, have kids been talking on the bus? If you can, find an opportunity to identify the source of their information and the extent of their knowledge. 'And then,' Hakanson says, 'very simply explain it. You might say, "Sex? That's a way to make a baby, but adults also do it to show love. Some people do it for a job."' She knows many parents find this conversation tricky. 'I'm a big fan of books, too. Talking to kids about sex is almost as hard as talking about divorce. You can even say, "That's a really good question. How about we talk about it on the weekend, and I'll find a book that talks about it more."' Hakanson's advice is the same whether a child is NT or ND – the only difference is perhaps a need, in some instances, to make the information more direct.

To parents who fear this conversation, or who are stuck working out the best age to start, Hakanson has this advice: 'Who do you want them to learn about sex from? Do you want them to get non-shameful, accurate information from you, or are you okay if they go and Google "sex"?' She says early and clear education also means that when other children are joking and giggling about it, knowledgeable children are less likely to become involved. It's also important in those cases when pornography is used to tease and torment children.

Hakanson says a difficulty in understanding body language or interpreting nuance means a neurodivergent child might not know whether someone likes them or is teasing them. Here, she suggests watching TV with your child, what she calls 'the lazy way to do sex education': 'But it's actually the most time efficient.

You might binge on *Gilmore Girls* with your child – whatever they want to watch. You might see a scene and say, "Do you think that they're flirting?" Because sometimes it can be really hard to tell if someone's flirting. A parent could then follow that up with, "I think they're flirting because …" and point out the language.' Of course, like any teen, they might ignore their parent, but it provides a lesson and a message that they can take on board.

Hakanson also offers advice about porn, which is being seen by school students, and being used to bully children. 'The best way to protect children is to have a conversation. Just having these conversations and talking about stuff actually protects kids, because you can't make an informed decision if you don't have any knowledge,' she says. 'Kids are turning to porn to learn about how sex works. It's the messaging that they get from sex which is problematic.'

THE POWER OF ONE FRIEND

Shared interests are a wonderful creator of bonds; they act as a friendship protector, allowing ND children to find comfort and grow alongside others. Attwood says one friend can make all the difference: 'Find a friend who is similar to you; sometimes it's another autistic person.'

'Theory of mind' is a concept that relates to the ability for a NT and ND person to read each other. And it goes two ways. 'Non-autistic people often can't read the blank face of the autistic person. But two autistic people often get on together in silence,' he says. Friendship might be two girls sitting beside each other drawing. 'They're not talking, they're not gossiping. They're not in-group, out-group. They're just drawing together. So that definition of friendship is just proximity and connection, but not a sense of rapport that others would expect,' he says.

Clubs, built around individual interests and passions, are crucial here. Robotic clubs. A school newspaper. Pokémon. Knitting. Drawing. Baking. Scouts. Birdwatching. Photography. Theatre. Gaming. Computer programming and design. Gardening. Jokes. Chess. Minecraft. Lego. Mini golf. Dungeons & Dragons. Trivia. Comic creation. The list is as long as individual children's passions and pursuits. From bagpipes and theatre to e-sports, coding and aviation. What is your child interested in? What drives their pursuits?

'It's essential to try and develop friendship on shared interests,' Attwood says. 'It's an opportunity for the autistic person to bring a sense of knowledge and value to the group.' Autistic girls, he says, often excel at the arts, and can sing in perfect pitch. A choir might be where they find belonging and friendship. Preserving wildlife is often another strong interest. 'Autistic girls can be phenomenal in their abilities with animals,' he says.

Many, but not enough, schools, do this well. One of those is St Peter's Lutheran College, a co-educational private school in Brisbane's west. Deputy head of college Lisa Delaney estimates thirty-five different clubs are available to students to capture the vast interests of the children. 'We've always been very good in allowing students to find their tribe; in creating opportunities for students to get together.' She says this has grown since Covid: 'We ran a number of different clubs and groups online for students, when we were in school at home.' Some of them – like the bagpipe group, for example, have flourished. Equally popular with all children, the clubs also allowed ND children to excel or find an interest in something outside the classroom, and they could participate at their own engagement level and speed.

While Delaney is clear in her view that awards aren't everything, the robotics club has fostered expertise that now sees children receiving awards for their work in the digital space. 'Those students are now getting to stand up in front of their peers, in front of their cohort, and receive commendations for the work they've done or the work they've put into something.' Delaney says the robotics program opened a 'world of opportunities' post-school, because it taught children to code and build robots, but they also used marketing and presentation skills that are not embedded in the class curriculum. 'It also allows neurotypical and neurodivergent students to work together with their strengths – and I think that's the winner. They should leave school thinking, "Okay, now I have all these opportunities because of school."'

> 'He has a great gang of buddies – they were at the same preschool, started school together, are mostly in the same soccer team.'

Clubs also help develop a sense of working together, being valued as part of something bigger, and a connection over a mutual passion. In the case of sport, it also delivers mentoring figures in coaches, club volunteers and parent helpers. 'In Australia, sportsmen are gods, and you don't challenge the gods,' Attwood says. 'But if you are in a team, there is also a team spirit and team members will support you.'

The connection between autism and humour is well-chronicled; Australian comedian, writer and actor Hannah Gadsby is one example. 'There is a connection between autism and humour,' Attwood confirms, 'especially stand-up comedy.' 'Neurodivergent people see connections that other people haven't noticed, and they become intoxicated by laughter. Laughter of the peer group is a drug. And they find this powerful and encouraging – their social challenges are accepted, they're a value to the group because they make people laugh.'

A sense of humour and an ability to deliver witty one-liners also stood out, particularly in ND high-schoolers, in helping to spark friendships. Sometimes, their quick wit was at the expense of a teacher, which prompted the label 'class clown', and also provided a connection to peers in class that endured over lunchtime.

Attwood says another component of autism is not seeing hierarchies. 'So, you're quite brave in making a comment to the school principal. And then you get extra status points by bringing the school principal down. In autism, that sense of humour – sometimes the ridiculous – is a natural process and can become popular with their peer group.'

Certainly, a strong sense of humour was an ND quality that surfaced many times in our research as a friendship protector, as did the physical size of the teen, particularly for tall autistic males. As one parent observed: 'We are very lucky in that he's currently six-foot two-inches, good looking and well spoken. If he gets bullied, he has absolutely no idea and just ignores it, so it goes away.'

Other attributes that build friendships include good listening skills. Buddy systems can help and so do role-playing conversations. Kaspar advocates the use of a child's strengths to guide their learning around friendship. She says a strength-based approach focuses on a child's abilities and knowledge rather than what they might lack. 'Sometimes people overuse or underuse certain strengths,' she says. 'So, for example, a child with ADHD might have a strength of zest. But when they're hyperactive, and they're jumping in everybody's face, that's the overuse of zest.' Framing it in a way that allows the child to feel good about themselves is important, so they think about managing their strengths, rather than seeing them as a deficit.

The use of 'signature strengths' or 'gifts of character' can help clarify what we care about and who we are, and this allows teens to flourish and deal with challenges. Kaspar nods to the twenty-four strengths categorised by positive psychology guru Martin Seligman, who organised them into six virtues – wisdom, courage, humanity, justice, temperance and transcendence. Children are able to use their own strengths to grow and to respond to challenges. Let's take the example of justice – the strengths sitting under that might be teamwork, fairness and leadership. It's a positive way to make sure all children understand, appreciate and use their strengths.

> *'In our house we call her autism her superpower. We celebrate it, and she has come to understand that her struggles with autism are similar to her sister's struggles with maths, or my struggle with weight loss – ha, ha!'*

Being able to repair friendships is also important, according to Turner. This is particularly the case for many ND teens who see issues in black and white, an inflexibility that can end friendship journeys prematurely. 'Bluntness is probably less of an issue from a social responsibility and friendship point of view,' Turner says. 'It's repair that is the really big thing.' He equates it to a partnership or family dynamic. 'If the goal is to never have arguments as a couple, good luck, that's just not happening. But if people can repair and come back together, things are okay.'

This stopped us in our tracks, because our research revealed a high proportion of ND children had lost friendships over something trivial. But if our teens – ND and NT alike – could be given the skills to 'repair' conflict and misunderstandings, a more fruitful friendship might ensue. Turner says practising conversations in a controlled environment could deliver good outcomes. Kids need to be taught how to approach someone and how the conversation might unfold – what to say and how to say it. This is no different to role-playing conversations with young children, and giving them the words to use in different situations. And while practising might not make things perfect, it can certainly provide skills to pop into that friendship toolbox that will contribute to a teen's happiness and mental health.

FRIENDSHIP TIPS FOR HIGH-SCHOOLERS

- The goal is quality over quantity. It's better to have one or two close friends than be a part of a big friendship group where you don't feel valued.
- Friendships are made in small moments. Seek out moments when there's just one or two people and strike up a conversation. Asking a question, or making a comment, is a good way to do that. It could be while you are waiting outside a classroom together or catching the same bus. Be brave and say something. If they ignore

you or are not interested, abort mission! Try again with a different person tomorrow. You won't be friends with everybody at school – you just need one or two friends you can trust.
- Finding friends is one thing but finding the right friends FOR YOU is another. Work on your friendship radar so you recognise what a healthy friendship looks like. Social researcher Dr Brene Brown created the 'Anatomy of Trust' to help us understand the seven elements of trust. She uses the acronym BRAVING which gives us all a great checklist:
  - **B**oundaries (Do they respect your boundaries?)
  - **R**eliability (Can you rely on them?)
  - **A**ccountability (Do they own their impact and take responsibility for things?)
  - **V**ault (Can you trust them with personal stories?)
  - **I**ntegrity (Do they do what they say they're going to do?)
  - **N**on-Judgemental (Can you be yourself?)
  - **G**enerous Lens (Do they give you the benefit of the doubt?).
- Don't put all your friends in one friendship basket. It's really smart to have friends outside of school. When we spend all day with people, it's normal that they'll get on our nerves sometimes. Having a second group of friends, or just one friend outside of school, is vital.
- The sooner you get comfortable communicating your personal boundaries, the better. Personal boundaries cover all aspects of our lives, including: activities ('I don't do horror movies'); privacy ('I'm not okay with you looking through my phone'); time ('I don't answer

messages after 9 pm'); and touch ('I don't do hugs'). Practise at home by saying: 'I'm not okay with …' or 'I don't do …' Boundaries are a way of communicating what you are comfortable with and are key to healthy friendships and romantic relationships.

- Struggling to find a group to sit with? Some groups are closed to newcomers, and that might have NOTHING to do with you. Once a group is calm, with no drama, some kids can be reluctant to rock the boat with new members. But there's nearly always a group at school who is happy to take new people in. Look for that group in your year level. And the other secret sauce of high school is to JOIN IN. Choose a club that you love and get involved. You'll regularly meet kids with similar interests, and it gives you somewhere to go at lunchtime.
- We all want a ride-or-die friend – someone who is fiercely loyal and is in our corner no matter what. But strong friendships take work. It's about showing up for people and giving them your time. If they have a basketball final on Saturday night, go to cheer them on. If they have a part-time job interview on the weekend, send them a message saying, 'You've got this!' If they get their heart broken, turn up at their house with ice cream, offer to watch a movie with them and keep them company. Strong friendships come from investing time and energy into other people, not simply responding with love-heart eyes on their Instagram posts.

4. SCHOOLYARD DYNAMICS

IMAGINE A GAME WHERE CHILDREN pretend they are signatories at an international conference, and they all represent a fictional country. The participants are given a card with the norms and rules of their country, as well as the things that would be insulting to them. In the country of Frownland, for example, it is polite to frown at people, stare hard into people's eyes to get their respect, and only say words that are utterly necessary. Smiling people, in Frownland, cause offence, as do casual conversations and people who gesture wildly when they speak. Over in Giggleville, the world is entirely different. Here, people giggle at everything, use their hands all the time, give very long answers and even hug people when you meet. Here, direct and abrupt answers are considered rude.

How would this game play out in a Year 3 class? Or a Year 5 class? It would create confusion, at the very least, but would also be upsetting for some. Author Kathy Hoopmann uses this example to explain autism to those who may not understand it; as well as to highlight how some people are insulted by other people's genuine attempts at friendliness. Needless to say, by the end of the game, it also demonstrates how similar people might gravitate towards each other.

Hoopmann has written more than twenty books, with translations into more than a dozen languages. Perhaps her best known are those about animals with a neurodivergence, including *All Cats Are on the Autism Spectrum, All Dogs Have ADHD* and *All Birds Have Anxiety.* But it is *The Essential Manual for Asperger Syndrome (ASD) in the Classroom,* that highlights how a cohort of children might understand difference by experiencing the world of difference. While the term Asperger's is no longer used, the lessons in Hoopmann's book are stellar.

In another example, Hoopmann suggests telling the story of three blindfolded men being allowed to touch an elephant for the first time. One touches the animal's side and imagines the elephant must be shaped like a wall. Another touches its trunk and thinks the elephant must look like a big fat hose. The third feels its tail, reminding them of a rope. Autism is a bit like only seeing one part of the elephant.

When a classmate arrives on crutches, peers can see that they cannot walk by themselves. They can see that they might need help navigating classroom tasks. With an unseen disability, it can be hard for children, particularly in primary school, to understand the world of the child who struggles in their group project, or who wants to play with them at lunchtime. However, a horde of lessons can be delivered to NT children about empathy, leadership and friendship, to help them better understand and value difference.

Hoopmann was first prompted to research and write about autism after a family member was diagnosed. But she could only find big heavy volumes with words aimed at doctors and psychiatrists – nothing aimed at children. She wanted something you could 'give to your next-door neighbour to explain a child's behaviour'. This led her to develop the characters in a series of books to help demystify autism for neurodivergent children.

But what about all of the NT children who fill their classrooms, playgroups and sporting teams? How do we ensure children understand each other, and the value of those who are different to them? How are autism and other neurodivergencies explained to the classmates who sit within a ruler's distance of them, all day every day, navigating maths problems and English comprehension?

In the past two chapters, we've seen how tough friendship can be for many ND children, but what happens when you put them into a classroom that is structured for NT learning?

For some ND kids it presents opportunities – new friends, new subjects and new lunchtime games. For others, it's a strange world where they feel they just don't fit – it's loud and busy and filled with bright lights and weird smells. Routines that shape their home life don't exist. Sometimes, it's difficult to read what others are saying to them. Perhaps their uniform hurts. They feel like they've been picked up and transported to another country, where the language and customs make everything difficult to understand. It's exhausting, even scary, they say.

> *'I am not like other kids but everyone expects me to be. I don't like the same things. I don't like clothes and shoes – they are so uncomfortable. I am always anxious and scared, and I don't know why, and I can't help it or control it.'*

Many of the educators in charge of the classroom don't understand them either. As one boy in Year 2 told us: 'I don't want to go to dress-up days because everybody, even the teachers, are different. I don't like it. It makes me sad, and the teacher tells me to just put headphones on and I don't like to do that, so why is she not listening to me say it?'

Or this from a girl, aged eleven: 'Teachers think I do everything wrong. Teachers make me write pages and pages and my hand cramps up and hurts. Teachers think I'm back-chatting when I ask them to explain why I have to do something.' Another girl in Year 4 agrees: 'I pretend that I am okay, but I am not okay every day, and I feel so sad but somebody else needs the teacher so I can't have her help me. My friends sometimes don't want to play with me.'

> **'I'm tired of having to pretend to be normal all day. It's exhausting.'**

Commonsense would dictate that a level of responsibility here, particularly in school settings that claim to be inclusive, falls on NT students too. 'They need to feel what it is like,' Tony Attwood says. Experiential learning by non-autistic peers of what it is like to be autistic might change others' behaviour. As one Year 12 biology teacher noted: 'One of my students, graduating today, is neurodiverse. He is persistent, resilient and extremely passionate about fossils. He has worked really hard and has excellent results. One day he said to me that he has to work hard every day to change his personality so he fits in and doesn't annoy other people, and it's exhausting for him.'

Inevitably, a curriculum-focus in high school has advantages for some ND students, who might have an interest in a particular subject. It might prove to be an avenue to meet like-minded peers who also share the same subject focus. But often, students can feel lost at high school, with multiple teachers in multiple rooms, and a timetable that changes each day. 'It's like a whole new universe,' says autism educator and author Sue Larkey.

The experience of a ND child is also shaped by the developmental age of their peers. 'In primary school, teachers teach students. In secondary school, teachers teach subjects,' says Larkey. 'If you met an English teacher, they'd say, "I'm an English teacher." Primary school teachers also teach English, but they'd never say, "I'm an English teacher."'

MASKING IN THE PLAYGROUND

High school can be experienced differently by boys and girls and is commonly the reason why girls are diagnosed with both autism and ADHD at an older age. Some girls will look and act just like everyone else, but not feel like anyone else. Experts use the term 'masking' or 'camouflaging' to explain this. Larkey says early criteria for the assessment of autism was male-based, and females presented differently, often going unnoticed. Often well-behaved and intelligent, they don't draw attention to themselves and work hard for that to be the case. But it means they are not offered support or assistance, and that, according to experts, can have strong consequences for both their confidence and motivation. This was confirmed by the parents we surveyed: 'My daughter masks heavily, so the child in class is not the child at home. Teachers often believe she's fine, but she's held everything in and is ready to explode.'

Indeed, during our research we often heard of young adult

women seeking their own diagnosis in the first year after leaving high school. They'd seen explanations of ADHD and autism on social media. 'I always felt a bit different. Now I know why,' one says. While a diagnosis might provide some comfort, it also points to lost years, with many girls having had to navigate their teens without any assistance.

Autism expert Michelle Garnett says that while both genders are believed to mask equally, girls mask more commonly across more settings and at a deeper level. 'So, it's more tiring and exhausting,' she says. 'And they do it because of what you think – to fit in, to fly under the radar … so they can avoid bullying, but also so they can make friends.' They believe if they can copy what someone else does, they can win a friend. 'It is sad to have to quash down their authentic self to be accepted,' Garnett says.

Garnett explains that girls have a stronger social motivation to make friends from an earlier age than boys overall, and difficulties fitting in to the 'teenage girls' set means a co-educational school is preferable for many. 'It's easier to make friends with boys, and there's research on that,' she says. Boys can have simpler demands, play less peer politics, experience less groupthink, and conflict can be resolved by walking away or moving on quickly. Friendships are often also around interests, including sport. That doesn't mean that ND boys have an easy ride though. Garnett says her clinical work showed boys can be 'pretty lonely and isolated in the teenage years' – often solid friendships came from shared interests with another male. Our research confirmed this.

In addition to camouflaging or masking to a greater degree across more settings, girls also tended to present with bigger mental health challenges. 'Both have mental health issues, but the girls tend to have very powerful presentations of anxiety and depression, with high levels of suicidality and self-harm,' Garnett says. Masking is exhausting and can lead to burnout. While Garnett's comments relate to autism, Autism Spectrum Australia says that most individuals with autism also have ADHD symptoms. Although, studies vary widely – some show the proportion of children with autism who also have clinical symptoms of ADHD is as low as fourteen per cent, while other studies suggest it is up to eighty-five per cent. Research also reveals that greater and deeper mental health issues are being experienced by girls with ADHD compared to boys.

Autism support specialist Kristy Forbes makes two additional points: firstly, we should remember there are other genders between binary male and female that need to be considered in this context. Secondly, while a girl might find it easier to pop into a library at lunchtime and read because she's frightened to be with people, our slowly changing male culture might mean alarm bells ring when a boy doesn't want to go and play football. 'So, it doesn't matter that he's autistic. It's just that he's not fitting into that stereotype. Girls might have more leeway.'

Psychologist Wesley Turner has worked with teen girls for a long time and encourages them to focus on their 'internal radar'. 'It's really about learning to get in touch with their gut feeling. These are not people who have intellectual issues – it's just that they haven't been shown, and haven't learnt how, to connect with themselves and trust themselves.'

Turner warns that masking could deliver long-term harm. He says we all act differently in different settings. For example, he would present differently watching football with his friends than he might during an interview. We all pick and choose when we shift into different presentations or different styles, depending on the circumstances. 'What happens with masking or camouflaging is that life becomes so complicated for people that they never get the opportunity, for a variety of reasons, to learn the difference between "this is who I *act* in different situations; and this is who I *am*."'

Turner works closely with ND teens so that they can learn what they like and want. He gives the example of a girl who wears make-up. She might hate it. It might feel horrible on her skin and make her sweat. He tries to get her to see herself camouflaging, by asking if she wears it for herself, or other people. Again, and this is Turner's mantra: 'It comes down to knowing yourself.'

Lisa Fife is head of Josiah College on the Gold Coast; a co-educational school where a primary diagnosis of autism is required for entry. 'Girls are more likely to care about being autistic. They don't want to be and they're expert maskers,' she says. 'They just want to fit in, especially when they hit those teenage years.' Fife sees daily how primary school-aged girls will 'remove the mask and they're happy to be themselves' but then 'puberty hits and on it goes again'. She says, a lot of work at Josiah College is put into that space around acceptance of self.

Larkey says a 'child who holds it together at school' might then have a meltdown when they arrive home. While some children mask, others might present differently in class. 'You might have a child and from the moment they walk in they're throwing bags, they're making noises, they're highly anxious,' Larkey says. Put yourself in the shoes of a teacher – they might have twenty-five other children, all with different personalities and challenges, strengths and weaknesses. In addition, those who are ND often have more than one diagnosis, as discussed earlier. Some children will be passive and not ask for help. Others are constantly asking for assistance and hitting the panic button. That puts a real burden on any teacher. But it also shows the complexity that umbrellas any one class of children.

THE POWER OF A FRIEND

One friend can make a world of difference. One friend can build a bridge across so many of the challenges attached to autism, in particular.

One friend.

This shouldn't be lost on teachers or parents of NT children; indeed, it represents a fabulous opportunity to develop leadership skills in children, simply by ensuring everyone has one friend or classmate. In many cases, the opportunity is delivered at school, through a buddy system, when a child first walks through the doors of a new classroom. 'I can't tell you how many times, in the diagnostic assessment of an adult, particularly with women, they say that their friend was "allocated" to them as a peer. That's the start of the friendship,' Garnett says. For all children, this presents a valuable opportunity to develop skills that will hold them in good stead for life.

'It's so powerful,' Garnett says. 'One friend. You only need one.' A single friend is able to provide a buffer; serve as a dam wall against the spectre of mental health issues, such as anxiety and depression, and can even prove more effective than a cohesive family. It can also change the balance in a classroom or group.

Our research confirmed that the act of one child sprinkling fairy dust across someone else's day could make an enormous difference. But the real power comes with allowing another child to believe in themselves. Some of the responses from parents, below, prove this point:

- 'A peer saw that my daughter had never received an award at school, so she made one for her – rewarding her for being the best and caring friend after my daughter had stood up for another student who was being bullied.'
- 'This year my son had a beautiful friend who is just super positive. When our son is negative, he will point out the positive or say what the reality is. For example, my son will say that his younger brother is a cheat, the friend will say, "I don't think he is a cheat, he doesn't understand the rules of the game."'
- 'He has an amazing little friend at school who will chat to him when he is melting down, or just give him some words of encouragement, or sticks up for him – because her parents have taught her about different people in the world.'
- 'The most heartwarming episode was when his Year 4 class went rollerskating. He was very out of his comfort zone and one of the boys took his hand and helped him skate around the rink. Ironically, this boy was quite a delinquent at school, but that day I saw the true measure of the young man.'
- 'At the beginning of the year, we were having trouble with getting our son to school due to high anxiety around having a new teacher for the year. One of his peers would come and meet us at the car and would talk with him and encourage him to walk into the school grounds with him. Having a friend by his side assisted with getting him back to school (on a reduced timetable to start).'

HOW TO TEACH CHILDREN THE VALUE OF DIFFERENCE

In *The Essential Manual for Asperger Syndrome (ASD) in the Classroom*, author Kathy Hoopmann suggests the following three activities for non-autistic children to learn about valuing difference in their peers. Whether delivered in the classroom or at home, these useful tips will help NT siblings, students and teammates better understand their ND peers.

1. Talk about how it would feel if you were doing something you loved, and then were suddenly moved and taken to a different world where nothing made sense. Have your children – at home or in class – write a story describing what happened and how they felt. If appropriate, use these examples to explain how an autistic child might feel each time they are forced to do something, or to go somewhere, when they are not ready or prepared.
2. Put a small piece of sandpaper somewhere where it rubs on your skin: perhaps in a sock. Then ask participants – teachers or students or friends – to sit on a small book unevenly. While that is happening, play repetitive annoying sounds, like scratching a chalk board. At the same time, have someone blow bubbles into the room while flicking the light switch on and off, over and over. How difficult would it be, in that environment, for a child to learn something new? 'I did that once for a bunch of teachers as well,' Hoopmann tells us. 'One lady, at the end, took out the sandpaper and ripped it up. She said it was the most horrible experience, but now she knew what some kids go through daily.'

3. Have children act out a scenario which includes the phrase: 'Come here.' Examples might include a monster wanting to eat little children, a mother wanting to give someone an ice cream, a teacher wanting to give an award, a bully wanting to hurt someone. Doing this highlights that children often know what someone means because of their facial expressions, hand gestures and body movements. Imagine how hard it would be, for many autistic children who only hear the words, and nothing else.

PART II: EDUCATION

5. FINDING THE RIGHT SCHOOL

IF YOU THINK IT'S HARD to imagine what an American college football coach, who had never coached an English soccer team before, could offer in the development of high-performance teams and positive culture, then you haven't seen the Apple TV+ show *Ted Lasso*. When the protagonist, Ted Lasso, is first recruited as head coach by the owner of a fictional English Premier Soccer League team – AFC Richmond – the lessons he delivers are as inspirational and uplifting, as they are profound. Wrapped up in the clever comedic script, viewers are reminded of the importance of setting the right tone for organisational success. Lasso, in his wisdom, promotes the team over the individual; the power of kindness; curiosity over judgement; vulnerability as strength. As Lasso demonstrates daily with his team, doing the right thing is never the wrong thing, courage is about 'having a go', as is unlocking the potential in others. He frequently refers to helping his team be the best versions of themselves – on and off the field – while at the same time encouraging them to work together to overcome challenges: 'You say impossible, but all I hear is "I'm possible".'

In school settings, the tone is also set from the top. Finding a school that is the right fit for your child is the single biggest issue facing families with a neurodivergent child. Our research revealed good and bad examples of both public and private schools, across primary and secondary schools. But the bad examples stood out largely because, as many parents explained, they were driven by academic outcomes and constant testing, school environments that prized conformity over individual pursuits, forced participation, teaching methods that did not acknowledge different learning styles, rigid timetables, high levels of bullying, poor understanding of inclusion and a lack of in-classroom support for teachers.

Psychologist Mary Kaspar raises a point we should all consider. She says it's not impairment that creates vulnerability, but 'rather the inequitable structures and systems which people with disabilities experience'. 'We know that neurodiversity presents challenges and goals for people in achieving what they want,' she says. 'So, yes, that needs to be managed but there also needs to be changes to the environment and how our culture thinks.'

'I've thought long and hard about this,' Michelle Garnett agrees. 'It's about embracing neurodiversity as the norm; not seeing it as "Oh my God, it's forty per cent or it's fifty per cent or whatever."' She believes the only way to tackle the issue is to create more awareness within schools and to challenge some of the underlying beliefs in society. 'What is neurodiversity? What does it look like? Can we teach that in classrooms? For so long, we didn't know much about the brain, and didn't talk about it, so it was believed if you looked the same as every other kid, you were the same as every other kid.'

With new knowledge, we should pivot. Garnett's plea is personal. For decades, neurodivergent (ND) children fell under the radar. 'I was one of them,' she says. 'We've come a long way, but I think there needs to be even more awareness.'

Parents, navigating a ND child's journey through the schoolyard and beyond, are experiencing numerous obstacles. 'Parenting a child who is ND is tough! Some days I feel like curling up in a ball and crying, but I have to continue advocating for my kid and helping him to be the best version of himself.'

'Primary school: ten out of ten. High school: zero out of ten. Hopeless'

Others are at their wits' end with a modern education system that claims inclusivity yet fails to deliver on promises. Parents who enrol their child into mainstream schooling should expect their child will be educated, safely. 'My biggest fear is I will end up on the front page of the paper because I've lost control, or my child has. If that happens, I want everyone to know how hard I tried to get help in a very broken system. Maybe not hard enough? But I am trying.'

Parents can see gaps in the system that should be providing for their ND child: 'There are billions of people in the world, all with different brains and different ways of learning, but our education system seems so narrowly focused on those who fit within the "normal" parameters. [The system] needs to be updated, more capable of adapting ... although I have no idea how this can happen!'

One of the biggest issues many parents face is getting the school to take their child's difference seriously. As one family noted: 'As parents we could see that the principal/diocese representatives did not believe the examples we had given them. They would see her, and as she wasn't throwing a chair across the room [they] would think she was "fine".' Others had a similar experience: 'She isn't enough of a problem for them, so they don't need to do anything to help her.' Another said: 'Where do you exactly want our kids to go when they are bright and polite but have slow processing speeds? Mainstream schools can't deal with that.'

> **'Mainstream schools don't have the resources or understanding to support my child and he doesn't meet the requirements of most special needs schools.'**

Some parents believed that schools were happy to have the academically gifted ND kids because it meant their national assessment scores would go up, but were less willing to adapt the environment to accommodate them. As a result, some parents were shopping around to find a better fit for their child. As one parent explained: 'We were at a state high when she was diagnosed, and when we talked to the guidance counsellor to ask how the school could support her, the counsellor asked what support we wanted. If you're new to this world, and you don't know, how can you know what will help? So, they offered nothing. When she had a suicide attempt, not one teacher or school staff contacted us or her. We tried distance ed, then homeschool, then Catholic school, then back to homeschool, where she pretty much does nothing due to burnout. No school helped in any way. Now this kid, who got straight As in primary school, hasn't completed Year 10.' Some families had more success: 'We have just changed to her fifth school. It is a small country school, and as the class sizes are small my child is getting much more teacher attention – so far this is translating into better grades.'

Many parents were frustrated by schools advocating inclusive values but failing to provide the support needed to be truly inclusive. As one mother said: 'Terrible! It is a private independent school. On paper they say they encourage diversity, but they would really prefer us to be elsewhere. The school routinely "manages children out" of the school and steers them to public schools. Honestly, my boy just has some trouble with maths and social relationships. He doesn't punch or kick or throw things.' Another attributed the issue to a 'lack of understanding, patience and time. Having an autistic child doesn't fit the mould of what schools celebrate. Seeing your child in a system that they aren't geared for is a soul-destroying experience.'

Of course, there are many exceptions, and they popped up in our research as families sang the praises of teachers, classrooms and whole schools that had worked in partnership with them and their child. Here, in general, families were supported by smaller class sizes, teachers who sought advice on how to engage their child, school wellbeing animals, and teachers who were either ND themselves, had children who were, or who had received training in teaching ND children.

These schools were spread across the public and private sectors, in city and rural areas, and in primary and secondary classes. 'Our state school has been absolutely brilliant,' one parent confirmed. 'She's in Year 8 and gets lots of support. I feel like her whole team really see her and know her and hold her.' Another parent had a similar experience: 'They keep the communication open. They teach children emotional regulation. On my son's first week, he came home and said, "Mum, my teacher sat down and asked me about me. She wanted to know me." Then another teacher on the playground asked him questions and welcomed him to the school. "Mum,

I love my new school," he told me.' Another parent had a similar experience. 'We are at a terrific school. I am a teacher there, and many of our teachers are ND or have ND children themselves. They operate on the belief that all children have the right to belong and that we need to change to support them. I know this is really rare.'

HOMESCHOOLING

Ironically, it was the experience with the education system that prompted so many parents to remove their child from school and educate them at home. Queensland Government data, released in November 2023, showed a twenty per cent increase on the previous year – with 10,048 registered homeschoolers (up from 8461) in that state alone. This increase can be attributed in part to the ability to access lessons online – and in many cases this is a choice parents made willingly.

There's no doubt that homeschooling across Australia has risen rapidly. In 2023 *The Guardian* reported the numbers of those enrolled in homeschooling had jumped 195 per cent between 2019 and 2023. While New South Wales had a 109 per cent increase, Western Australia, South Australia and Victoria also had increases of more than seventy per cent. The pandemic provided an impetus for many families to make the decision to homeschool. In many cases, as our research has also shown, this was a result of children being ND and struggling to learn or enjoy class.

Some parents relish the role of teacher and noticed their child thriving: As one parent said: 'I feel homeschooling has eased our stress and my son has made great gains in many areas just by having a caring and supportive environment. I have seen him go from an anxious, stressed and angry child to a quiet, beautiful and chatty little boy. I'm so proud of him.'

Many others turned to homeschooling as a last resort after repeated attempts at different schools failed. In some cases, this meant giving up their jobs to homeschool, which had both social and economic consequences for the whole family. In addition to the increased burden of less money coming into the home, some parents also found the experience isolating, and missed out on interacting with colleagues and opportunities for promotion.

The reasons behind families eschewing a mainstream education or making the decision to withdraw their child varies widely. For some families, their child faced playground bullying. Others recognised that the school was under-resourced – they felt their child was invisible in a large class group or the teaching staff lacked an understanding of neurodivergence. As one parent said: 'There are some amazing teachers out there and there are some very terrible ones, including principals who won't do anything about the bad behaviour of some other kids. I don't see my child going back to school at this point.'

Rigid rules and a lack of understanding from staff means that some ND students are being left behind: 'School – the work – doesn't make sense. I don't understand what the teacher is telling us. I don't want to ask questions and I don't know what I need to ask. I can't remember when things are due. Or where to find things. We use different platforms. I forget. I can't concentrate on class. And I don't have many friends. It's very lonely.' For some ND kids, the school environment is the most challenging they will face: 'Outside of school I don't feel as different, people are understanding, I can interact with people who are accepting, I feel safe. I only feel like I have a disability at school.'

Parents perceive that the school system does not value, or sometimes doesn't even see, the difference between students. As one parent noted: 'We ended up homeschooling at [the school's] suggestion, which is very difficult as a working single parent. The school put so much pressure on us to attend and then left them in an office, so it's not about learning, it's about ticking boxes for the department.'

IS THE EDUCATION SYSTEM FAILING OUR KIDS?

One of the biggest issues for the parents we surveyed is that all schools are part of a larger education system that delivers a national curriculum and operates under set policies, rules and goals. Many parents see a system failure in how inclusion is practised and describe an old education framework that is trying to reboot to function in modern times. As one parent told us: 'Our schooling system is broken. Archaic behaviour management approaches are often utilised for ND students, which are harmful and not effective. ND kids don't respond to sticker charts and external reinforcers. The ability to get help for our kids is a privilege in this country and it should be a fundamental right.'

Andrew Whitehouse, a Professor of Autism at the Telethon Kids Institute and the University of Western Australia, is widely considered a global autism expert. He is also on the National School Resourcing Board, which oversees school funding models. In his view: 'We've got a twenty-first century view of disability and neurodiversity working within nineteenth century infrastructure, and twentieth century levels of funding, and it simply doesn't fit. We're going to need generational shift firstly, in terms of funding. Teachers and education systems are extremely stretched, and every dollar is fought for with ferocity. And so, we need to ensure that if we are going to actually provide education that accords with our twenty-first century view of humanity, we need to fund schools appropriately. And really, is there any better investment in our country than helping kids thrive within schools?'

This view of introducing a more modern and flexible approach to learning is supported by parents of ND kids, who first experienced a change to the school system during Covid, when many schools had to adopt digital learning models. What they realised was that even basic lessons that were delivered during that time have been lost in a rush to return to how things have always been done. As one parent told us: 'That flexible lesson delivery helped many kids, especially ND kids. Schools promised they'd carry those lessons forward. That has not happened.'

> '[The school] developed some inclusive policy but this does not yet translate to action on the ground [due to] lack of resources, knowledge, experience and unconscious bias and ableism.'

The shift Whitehouse is advocating for is witnessed daily by parents. For their neurodiverse child, one parent told us, attending mainstream school is like fitting 'a square peg in a round hole'. Another parent noted: 'Schools still use a medical model of trying to "fix" the child to be more neurotypical. As much as my daughter masks, all I hear is "she is fine at school". In reality, she is running a treadmill every day and comes home and collapses into a heap.' Yet another parent attributed part of the systemic problem to a lack of staff training. 'I am a teacher and I see in all schools they don't have the ability to respond to ND children because they don't live the experiences some parents do. They don't understand that these kids don't have a choice.'

Professor Linda Graham, director of the Centre for Inclusive Education at QUT, says much of the focus in schools is on how to get ADHD students to pay more attention in class. 'That's actually asking them to do something that they find difficult to do,' she says. A child unable to walk is not encouraged to walk better; a ramp was usually built, she says. 'Everything we do is based on the social model of disability, and the concept of barriers and adjustments. The problem with ADHD is that because people think it's not a disability, these kids tend not to get adjustments.'

Graham says schools need to consider 'design pedagogy and assessment so that they get rid of the barriers that are going to trip these kids up in the first place'. Simple examples included teachers providing repetition, checking comprehension regularly and issuing instructions in brief sentences. 'No soliloquies,' she says, 'where they just tell kids to do five things and then wonder why they've only done one. They need to provide solid, tangible and written support so that once those instructions have left the kids' working memory, they've got something to refer to. Teachers need to use visual supports and limit distraction. They need to build in pauses in the way that they teach.'

Kristy Forbes is an autism support specialist who is autistic, has ADHD, is a teacher and homeschools her children. The most common question she is asked, in relation to education, is: 'How do I get my child to go back to school?'

The reasons a child might not be at school are complex – driven by suspensions, expulsions or something termed 'school refusal' or 'school can't', where a child simply can't navigate a path to attending school for a variety of reasons. Many ND families report this as a challenge for their child. Clinicians also saw a jump in the number of students resisting school post-Covid.

'I don't have a simple answer. But usually, it's taking some time to really hear the experience that the family has had.' Almost always parents want their child to receive a good education, to have a healthy sense of self and to be safe. 'And that doesn't always mean being in a school,' she says. 'I live in the grey. And I would never say, "This is the right way or that is the right way," but certainly it's imperative that we have options, not alternatives, to mainstream school.'

Forbes is concerned about the lack of professional development for teachers and awareness across the board. 'How can we give a blanket statement of inclusion when we don't know who we're working with or supporting? I might say I'm trauma informed as a professional. But what if I have a client who's experienced something I'm out of my depth with? That doesn't mean I'm trauma informed in that moment. So, inclusion means that we address the individual in front of us, and we make their right to an education accessible.'

Forbes says many parents are feeling shame because they are being gaslit. 'It's the blaming and the shaming of parents – telling mothers their child is anxious because they are. We haven't shifted if we're still placing blame. And I don't want to be hard, but the ignorance involved with giving someone such belittling information is so unhelpful.' She argues that in these situations, autistic people have to become the teachers, guiding educators and healthcare professionals to understand better the world of those in front of them.

TOP OF THE CLASS

At some schools, in specialist settings, the classes are built around the needs of the students. At Josiah College on the Gold Coast, autism needs to be the primary diagnosis for entry. All classes are capped at ten students and are overseen by a teacher and a teacher's aide. While the Australian curriculum is taught, there is no homework or competitive sport, windows are glazed, noise kept at a minimum and the lighting is soft. The air conditioning is silent and there are myriad small spaces across the campus to accommodate students outside of class. Swings are also built outside each classroom; the emergency alarm – a slow drumbeat – was chosen by the children who begin each day with exercises to the music they choose. Visual timetables are featured on walls, along with big posters illustrating a measuring beaker where children can label – and change – how they are feeling through the day.

'They don't have to say anything because that can be hard. They just do it,' says Simone Kiprioti, the college's senior school dean. At this school, teachers move between classes, not children. Take-Five cards, when a child needs a break, are provided to students, and teachers can also hand them out. At lunchtime, there are Pokémon clubs and mentor programs, ping-pong tables and basketball hoops. Laptops remain at school, and in recognition that it is often hard to have a child up and out early in the morning, there is a soft starting time each day. On the day of our visit, the children are told school will finish at lunchtime on Friday, meaning they can leave at midday. The chorus of disappointment is unmistakable; they don't want to leave early. 'Can I stay?' one asks. A second suggests it's in his school contract that he gets to stay until the afternoon bell.

Lisa Fife, head of Josiah College, says her aim is for each

child to reach their full potential. 'There's so much inside every child and when people make assumptions about what they can and can't do, and don't give them an opportunity to try, it's devastating.' In 2024, the school had ninety pupils and a growing waiting list for students from Prep through to Year 11. 'There aren't a lot of options for students on the spectrum who don't have a cognitive deficit, but can't cope with a mainstream setting,' Fife says.

While kids at Josiah are being taught the same curriculum as mainstream schools, Kiprioti says, 'We're stripping away all of those stresses that occur in other settings.' Smaller classroom sizes allow teachers to 'be more flexible and scaffold exactly where they need to'. Such is the success of Josiah, that it is now acting as the model for other communities planning similar education facilities. But it also raises the question of access: both the expertise and costs required to set up and run specialist schools, as well as the associated fees for parents.

The demand, though, is certainly there. Take Reverend Dr Ann Edwards, an Anglican priest who is also a speech pathologist, researcher and parent of an autistic child. Edwards has also been diagnosed with ADHD. She is behind a new Brisbane kindergarten that is now being planned. 'Parents are just trying to navigate these systems, trying to find the right services,' she says. Many are lost when they come up against big cumbersome structures that don't advocate for the individual. The transition to school for autistic children is difficult and a kindergarten that equips them for a long educational journey is a game-changer. Edwards says a neuro-affirming framework, where individual differences are encouraged and valued, will underpin the new school. Staff will include a special education teacher, speech pathologist and occupational therapist, who will be supported by therapists that individual families might access outside the school gates. This is a vote-winner for many families because, in some schools, individual therapists are banned; schools don't allow entry – despite it being recommended by many experts.

'I think what we are trying to do is to vaccinate [parents] against any idea that the child has the problem,' Edwards says. Her hope is they leave kindergarten having experienced 'success in a classroom setting and knowing that they can learn'. Teaching the language of school – how class routines work, as well as how to find their calm space and recognise when and how to ask for help – is a critical first step. 'We'll explicitly teach those skills before they walk into a classroom,' she says. Parent and medical referrals will help with entry, but Edwards says local schools have already shown interest in referring families.

TIPS FOR ADVOCATING FOR YOUR ND CHILD'S EDUCATION

While select specialist schools are focused on preparing students and their families for learning and a workplace that might follow, most parents have no idea of what to expect from the mainstream school system, how their child will respond to school, or their role in advocating for their child. Speech pathologist Dr Bronwyn Sutton describes four levels of advocacy that are key to a ND child's success at school:

1. Parental advocacy starts by teaching parents and carers how to have focused and respectful meetings. 'For

parents, I would suggest a meeting with the teacher once a term, which is scheduled with an agenda, and to continue these meetings all the way through from Prep to Year 12,' says Sutton. 'Parents need to be taught and supported to become advocates, because they're going to be advocates for the child all the way through their school years.'

2. Teacher advocacy involves educating and coaching teachers so they can advocate for the child to the parent, but also within the school system. 'I know every other kid needs to sit on the floor at assembly. But for this kid, let's make an exception. So that's the second level of advocacy.'

3. Systemic advocacy is where parents 'meet with the principal and actually look at what's happening from a whole-of-school point of view'. A student's team might be made up of an occupational therapist, speech therapist and psychologist, as well as the primary support person for that child. 'What can be done from a whole-school point of view?'

4. The most important advocacy comes from the ND child. 'So, we start teaching them from a very young age to self-advocate,' Sutton says. AI offerings, such as ChatGPT, have been a major player in this space because it means a child of five can write a 'very respectful email to their parent, teacher or principal to advocate for themselves'. (The use of AI was brought up repeatedly by experts; many saying it will offer a child the way to put numbers or sentences together and allow teaching efforts to be directed at more social learnings.)

HOW TO CHOOSE THE RIGHT SCHOOL

Knowing how the school system works – from their first day through to graduation – is an important first step in choosing the right school for your child. How a school operates is important to a child's comfort level, and our survey revealed an overwhelming difficulty for kids transitioning from primary school to high school. As many parents noted, their child's experience deteriorated as their school years advanced: 'I have been a teacher for twenty years. My boy started high school this year and it has rocked my world how very difficult we find mainstream schooling. There are very limited options for ND children.' All of a sudden, a child who has had one teacher each year in the same classroom, will have seven or eight different teachers and have to find half a dozen classrooms across a school campus within a short timeframe. It can be mayhem for many.

Psychologist Wesley Turner says it is important for children to feel as secure as possible. Parents might consider taking them for walks around the school during the holidays, before they start, so they can locate the toilets, the library and the tuck shop, for example. Providing a map might help, so kids can walk through how their school day is likely to play out. 'Pre-scaffolding predictability' is invaluable, Turner says. 'When you prime people, they find it easier to cope.'

Part of the issue with the modern education system is that many of our old classroom practices have been upended. 'At school, in years gone by, you tended to sit at a desk, you received information from the teacher, and you regurgitated that information during exams,' says autism expert Tony Attwood. The teacher passed on the information for students to digest. Now the emphasis is on group work, in which a large table of children are expected to interact. 'The problem is that when you assess a person this way, social difficulties can get in the way of learning. When we look at an autistic individual, often their best way of learning is solitary, or one-on-one, either via a computer screen, a book, or individual tuition. The moment you get multiple voices and a social dimension, it takes more brain effort than the actual academic task itself,' Attwood says.

Sue Larkey advises parents to go with their gut instinct when picking the right school environment for their child. 'If you turn up and think this school isn't for my child, don't try it. Walk away. Parents need to trust themselves because so often parents will say to me, "I knew it. I knew it from the first visit."'

This can be difficult because we all make mistakes, and parents often lack confidence when their child is starting school. In many cases, a diagnosis is made mid-way through schooling. Larkey says to consider the 'whole school'. Don't base a decision on Kindergarten or Prep, because often, they are 'set up for our diverse learners', with more routines and structure in place. 'Go look at a Year 3 class, a Year 6 class, because your child is going to be at the school for seven years,' she says. Consider the school's learning support offerings, too. 'Is there a dedicated person you can build a relationship with?' That person could be more important than the classroom teacher, who changes each year. 'You need someone there to be an advocate for your child.'

Author and psychologist Dr Mary Kaspar asks this question: 'If you really want to shortcut an approach, look at how they treat the most vulnerable people.' This could be evident in the school's anti-bullying practices, for example, or in a clear code of ethics. 'If you go into a school, you get a sense of it,' she says. How does it operate? How do people talk to each other? How is it structured? Is there an over-focus on competition or awards?

Dr Michelle Garnett recommends parents get a sense of how

inclusive the school feels. 'Are the kids being mean? How do they treat a stranger in the mix? Because your kid is going to be a stranger in the mix,' she says. 'They always say it takes a community to raise a child and it's so true, and it's especially true if that child is ND.'

Professionals are also an important part of your advocacy team – will the school welcome the advice of outside experts recommended by families. 'If everyone is working together – the professionals, parents and teachers – the child is going to do so much better, because of that alliance.' Garnett adds another factor in choosing a school. A good school, she says, is evidenced by happy kids and low levels of expulsion and exclusion. She says support groups and social media groups – word of mouth – can also be invaluable. Finding others who have walked your path can clear it, sometimes, by telling their own story.

WHAT TO LOOK FOR WHEN CHOOSING A SCHOOL FOR YOUR ND CHILD

- Seek recommendations from other families and online discussion groups where people have experience at the school you are considering. Connect with those parents and ask questions.
- Don't just visit Kindergarten, Prep or Year 1, try and visit an older school class and see how students treat each other and interact with their teacher. Early school years are more inclusive and cater to diverse learning experiences, so this is not always the best guide.
- Read the school newsletter. That's where you'll pick up on the values the school promotes. What children are

being recognised regularly, and for what?
- How does the school say it practises inclusivity? This might show up in the type of student awards they advocate, the support unit it boasts, the service opportunities on offer, the anti-bullying policy and how it is implemented, or the school's ethics statement.
- Look at the options for in-school and extracurricular clubs, teams and activities that the school offers and how these align with the interests of your child. Being able to engage with like-minded people helps ND and NT children to appreciate each other's strengths and differences, which can positively influence how they perceive friendships in and outside the classroom.
- Don't dismiss your gut instinct. You know your child better than anyone. Value that.

6. THE POWER OF A TEACHER

Have you ever had a teacher who changed your trajectory – a teacher who took you aside and made you see something in a different light? A teacher whose own journey resonated with you and gifted you a real sense of optimism? A teacher whose care started with the curriculum but ended with capturing your heart and soul?

While the curriculum is what a teacher *must* deliver, care is what they *can* deliver. All teachers have the power to capture the mind of each student in front of them and deliver a gift that can last a lifetime. There is no difference between neurotypical (NT) and neurodivergent (ND) children; every child will respond to a teacher who makes time to understand them. But for ND children, this might be harder for a number of reasons – they might be masking during school hours or not be able to communicate in the way other students do. They might act out their fears and appear naughty or disengaged. They might be chaotic, with their belongings a mess. Some might be incredibly studious and quiet. Some might want to answer every question while others might answer none. They might have an all-consuming interest in one subject, and no interest in others.

Lisa Fife, head of Josiah College, says the power of a teacher is difficult to measure. A child can spend more waking hours with an educator than a parent, and the relationship should be underpinned by trust.

Simone Kiprioti, who is senior school dean at Josiah College, agrees. She says a teacher's power is delivered by the connection they are able to forge with a child: 'It's all about relationships. That's what makes a good teacher. Full stop.' She tells new staff that building a bond with their autistic students is the first and primary focus for them, because this is what their success will be based on. 'It's almost like newborn imprinting because our kids have rigid thinking. If the first thing the teacher does is something they don't like, then it's really hard to unpick that.'

At Josiah College, individual teachers spend time, before a child starts, getting to know their likes and dislikes – a privilege afforded to teachers at a college with a small numbers of students. Kiprioti admits 'this would be an idyllic world for every school and every teacher'. Fife says the gold star is a teacher who can empower a child to the point where 'they understand themselves, and where they can speak for themselves and say what they need and are happy to say what they can and can't do. That is paramount.'

Not every teacher can deliver such an outcome; it is a skill and a gift that is often undervalued. Fife believes that there are many well-qualified teachers 'who know all the theory' but do not necessarily 'have the passion, the patience or the heart'. Then there are those who might not hold specific ND qualifications but have 'a real passion for working with children, who are in a learning support setting or who are considered the underdog, and they just love teaching'. That latter group throw their efforts and energy at finding out what works for each child.

Most teachers believe that inclusion is important. But where it gets tricky, says educator and author Sue Larkey, is in their ability to deliver. Three hurdles often stand in their way: time, resources and support. 'They want more time to actually do training. They can't even get released to do PD (professional development) since Covid. It's ridiculous,' she says. They also want time to meet with the parents of a child. 'A five-minute parent-teacher interview isn't going to be enough if you have a ND child in your class.'

Secondly, they want the resources to do their job properly. 'There's no other profession where you have to pay for your own training and resources,' Larkey says.

Thirdly, it is difficult for a teacher to support a child if they feel unsupported themselves. Imagine, she says, if a teacher who had to deal with a particularly tricky day was given a small care pack at the end of the day. 'We don't budget for anything like that, and as a result, some teachers will then take a sick day or actually just stop trying.'

This feeds into the wider community narrative about the value of teachers. 'I often say to parents, "Would you have thirty children in your house?" They respond by saying their child wouldn't cope. But we are asking your child to cope in a room with thirty other children five or six hours a day.'

Autism expert Michelle Garnett is also not critical of teachers; she believes our schools are packed with good educators who work in a big unwieldy system that is often valued – and judged – on academic merit and uniformity.

A school's culture in its commitment to inclusivity also depends on the school principal or head, who sets the tone for staff. Those staff who were ND or who had a ND child stood out in our research for their empathy, but also their ability to change their classrooms and teaching strategies to benefit *all* students.

Many teachers have received no training in different learning pathways, which begs the question of how schools can then market what they offer as an 'inclusive education'. While some of the current classroom practices are outdated – such as reward charts – other teachers are spending their own money to bring in resources that might help a child in their class. Others are funding degrees and courses out of their own pockets so that they can better understand each of the children in their class. And many of them told us how some parents, too, eschew the idea of a label and will not – despite gentle prodding – seek an assessment for their child. That can be frustrating for a good educator, who wants each student to reach their full potential.

As one teacher told us: 'Relationship building is important and he's making better choices in the classroom. [But] outside in the playground, all the wheels fall off. His parents don't want to hear anything, although I've never mentioned any word that begins with "a" ... *Rain Man*, the movie, did immeasurable damage. My own child is autistic and he loves being neurodivergent!'

Another teacher had experienced similar issues: '[Tom] is a boy without a diagnosis. He is oblivious to the world around him and has lots of vocal tics and some stims. He's academically able when you can support his lack of executive functioning to get to the right class with the right materials and is able to start a task. He can't work in a group and struggles to work alongside others. He loves Lego and battleships and eats a wonderful lunch every day, but by himself or with me, for safety, as he's teased and ridiculed.'

We heard numerous examples of teachers going out of their way to help their students: '[Adrian] is undiagnosed. Every speech therapist and occupational therapist has recommended his parents seek an evaluation. They do not want the label. My day wavers between allowing him to play all day whilst the rest of the class participate in learning, to providing myriad adjustments to get him to join in one task.'

Many are learning on the job: 'I love the way the little one in my kindergarten class sees the world differently to others. He seeks reassurance that all is well with the world using the sweetest phrases and safe conversations. He is blossoming now and branching out of his safe words and conversations and beginning to have less meltdowns if things are a bit different. He's taught me a lot about ensuring we can prepare little people for how things may change through the day.'

TEACHING WITH HEART

Our research threw up some truly dreadful examples of how ND students were taught within the school system, and this was across all sectors – public and private – with examples in both city and regional areas. We also heard some stunning examples of teachers who successfully engaged with a child who was struggling. In one case, for example, a teacher bought a fishing tackle box with her own money and took it into school as a gift for a student. She understood her student loved fishing and used his interest and passion as a way of teaching him to organise his belongings. It worked a treat. The examples of clever and novel ideas run to pages, but here are a few we've chosen in a bid to show how some teachers are successfully engaging some of their ND students.

- 'At the moment, my son's teachers are organising for him to record his voice for the local train to celebrate the International Day of People with Disabilities. Some of his friends are going to go on an excursion to listen and celebrate him.'
- 'The science teacher at high school this year was aware of his difficulties in taking notes, writing in general, and keeping up in class. So, they printed off a booklet of the lesson slides but omitted key points that he then had to fill in as the lesson proceeded in an attempt to engage him throughout the lesson, rather than having him become discouraged with his inability to keep up.'
- 'A beautiful inclusion support team organised a visit to the local creek once a week during their lunch hour. It gave the kids a space where they felt seen, heard, responsible and relaxed. They even ended up participating in a puddle jumping competition one year!'
- 'Primary school set up a fake camera outside my son's classroom in Year 2 to stop him running/leaving class and attempting to just go home. He was obsessed with CCTV at this time and was convinced the principal could see, so never left class again.'
- 'Classroom teacher has provided a comfort entry to class. My daughter becomes overwhelmed starting the day; the teacher allows her to spend ten or fifteen minutes in classroom before bell to adjust to the environment.'
- 'This year, his teacher has given him and a few others in the class "Recharge Cards". They can hand them in at any time of day and get ten minutes to recharge. This can be ten minutes on the iPad, playing with Lego, doing physical exercise. This has been a game-changer, as he is in charge.'

- 'Her Year 5 teacher wrote her a card at end of year and thanked her for everything she taught him that year.'
- 'A beautiful English teacher recognised that he couldn't bring himself to speak up in class to ask for help, so developed a plan that he was to email her in class and send his work via OneNote for feedback.'
- 'Teacher emailed me today to let me know there is a fire drill scheduled for Monday after recess, so I can spend the weekend prepping her.'
- 'One teacher told the kids he couldn't spell and probably had dyslexia right from the start. He got the kids that could spell to correct his; he included everyone and he made learning (especially maths) super fun and active (including ball throwing while learning).'
- 'The teacher started a communication book just between my son and her. She writes questions or thoughts in there and leaves it on his desk. When he feels like it, he responds and often asks something back. He felt genuinely connected but with zero demand.'
- 'My son was part of a musical theatre group as a kid and the teacher who ran it just saw a spark in him and gave him a lead role in Year 2. This was such a game-changing experience for him and gave him such a sense of self-worth and confidence. He's been singing and acting ever since.'

One teacher we spoke to brought caterpillars into her class from her own garden. Another allowed a student to perform his poetry slam at whatever point in the day he wanted. Later she asked about his anxiety/stress level doing the performance. He rated it as a two out of ten, compared to the apprehension in the lead-up, which he said was nine out of ten. 'Then they talked about anticipation being worse than the actual event.' This same teacher was very structured, communicated continually with parents and offered breaks and 'jobs' outside the classroom when she saw the same child reach a certain point. 'He would never have performed poetry slam previously,' his mother says.

> *'One teacher made a jar filled with water and glitter for [my son] to use when he was feeling frustrated; another introduced him to fidget toys.'*

In another case, the teacher bribed a student to get their work done with trips to the school cafe, which the student loved. And in another, the teacher got to know the student, before telling his parents that he had a real talent for computer programming. 'This made me cry because up until that point all feedback about his learning had been negative,' his mother says. 'I felt like none of his teachers could look past his learning difficulties and see the intelligent kid I knew him to be.'

A music teacher told us about a student who was obsessed with Marvel and Star Wars. 'They've started composing film scores and are now applying to study composition at tertiary level. They've come a long way from being very anxious about everything. They recently said music has changed their life forever.'

PUNISHMENT VS REWARDS

It would be remiss to skip over the bad examples of how some ND kids are being treated in schools. We need to see these and call them out, in a bid to stamp them out. It is clear that a lot of teachers have not received any recent training or professional development and lack an awareness about neurodivergence. As a consequence, some teachers don't have the skills to educate a ND child. Reward charts were possibly the worst example, as one parent described: 'In this class a teacher would give points if students did jobs or completed lessons. The points could be used to go to the bathroom, have an early mark or get prizes. This day the teacher set an activity for the student to do. My son didn't understand what to do. He couldn't ask his friends because they would both get in trouble. He tried asking the teacher but he was told to do it himself. He tried but was getting nowhere, so stopped. As he was sitting there, he started to feel that he needed to go to the toilet, a feeling he gets when he is nervous. The teacher said no points, no toilet. So, he ended up soiling himself in class.'

Other parents reported similar issues with reward systems: 'In Year 1 they would have a shared reward chart, so the class would all get a prize if they did things on time as a collective. One time they had to pack up their activity and put the equipment in their school bag and then get back to the mat. My son didn't make it within the time and all the other kids were already on the mat. The whole group was penalised and missed out on the reward. He said all the kids were screaming at him and called him dumb. He said it was awful and cried about it at night for over a week.'

These weren't the only examples of reward charts being used; a disciplinary tactic that angered, frustrated and saddened experts who work with ND children. 'It gives me the shivers,' Garnett says. She knows a teacher might have good intentions, but this 'stick and carrot, dog-training misbehaviour modification' has no role in the classroom. 'It might work for dogs, but we are not dealing with dogs. You can get a dog to do anything for food. That's not the case for an autistic person, because we're more complex than that,' she says.

In another case, an education assistant says she worked in a classroom with a six-year-old autistic child who also had ADHD. 'I have seen a teacher stand in front of [him] to stop him from leaving a classroom when he was dysregulated. She stood in front of him growling for him to go and sit down. He ended up pushing past her and getting suspended again for assaulting a teacher. Our educators are underpaid, unsupported, (and) under-educated about teaching students with disabilities.'

In other examples told to us by parents:

- 'Principal pulled up some photos of meth addicts on his computer. Showed them to my son and said: "If you make bad choices, you end up like these people ... so that's why we need to make good choices." He was only in Year 5 at the time!'
- 'My daughter's special interest is reading. She snuck in the back door of the school library (her safe place) then was forcefully dragged out by two staff members as she went through the wrong door. My daughter's education asisstant quit, because being a receptionist pays more ...'
- 'My son calls out answers as he's super excited to know them. He is constantly being moved due to yelling out. The teacher recently dropped him from extension for yelling out an answer and standing up out of excitement.'
- 'When I told my seven-year-old's Prep teacher two years ago that we were going down the route of an ADHD diagnosis, she laughed in my face and said, "She doesn't have a behavioural issue, she has a working memory issue."'

- 'My daughter has permission to have fidgets with her, but one teacher threatens to throw them in the bin if my daughter plays with them.'
- 'My son said the class was tasked to be creative and draw a spider. He drew all six legs on one side. In front of the whole class the teacher said, "Don't be so ridiculous, what are you in Year 3 or something?" He was in Year 5, and that being said in front of the whole class destroyed him.'
- 'He was called "dysfunctional" by one teacher, a "coward", a "disappointment" and a "disgusting little boy" by another, and then the last one we complained about referred to him as "a waste of space" and hit him over the head with some paperwork he had in his hand.'
- 'Kids stuck a Sticky Note on his back; [when] he asked around everyone said no. He then went up to the teacher and she even said there was no Sticky Note on his back!'
- 'A child smacked my son in the head. My son told the teacher, and he was told to ignore it. Kids did it again. My son started to cry. The teacher told him to "harden up and stop being such a crybaby". When I confronted the teacher and principal, I was told, "Hurt kids, hurt kids". So, nobody is held accountable and my kid suffers for it. Same kid broke my child's arm a week earlier. Didn't even get a detention. My son told that kid the next day to "F**k off and leave me alone". The school suspended him for four days for using foul language.'

FORGET THE APPLE, TEACHERS NEED SUPPORT

While none of the examples above are excusable, it's important to put this in context. The reality is that many teachers are over-worked, under-resourced and under-valued. 'All families have good and bad classroom stories – that's life,' one parent said. 'Schools are doing their best. Some do better if they have more support and access to specialists and extra teacher aides.' Another said: 'I find the teachers are generally excellent, however they are overstretched and unsupported, they need more hands-on help in the classroom.'

While many parents had a better experience at public schools, others said staff resourcing was a higher priority at private schools. Class sizes also vary widely across the education sector, as does the experience and knowledge of teachers.

Larkey doesn't mince words. 'We have a big problem in Australia,' she says. On average, a teacher stays in the job for five years and often their decision to leave is prompted by student behaviour. Many universities do not value educating teachers about neurodiversity or provide strategies that might help them engage all learners. She says: 'I started off as that teacher who learnt nothing about autism, had a child with autism in my class and was heartbroken. I didn't know how to educate him,' she says. Three decades later, she has this question: 'How can we have this systemic problem that teachers are only staying for five years, and yet we are not addressing this at the university level?'

So, what should a university education in this area look like?

Larkey answers without taking a breath. 'Proactive practical strategies that actually help teachers know how to set up their classroom, how to understand neurodivergent children, and how neurodivergent children need to be taught differently.' The bonus, she argues, is that most of these strategies worked for the whole class. 'For example, this is a very anxious generation, so putting in place routines … when you make it less overwhelming for the ND child, you're actually making it less overwhelming for everyone,' she says.

Professor Linda Graham, director of The Centre for Inclusive Education at QUT in Brisbane, says universities differ. 'There's all this stuff about education students needing more time in schools – but in this particular area, that's not going to help because schools themselves don't know what to do. They need a very solid grounding in understanding how students learn. And how some students are different to others.'

Once upon a time, classrooms were bare. Now they are full of colours and sounds – sensory distractions that can make it difficult for some learners. Open-plan classrooms can also present a challenge. Professor Tony Attwood says while there are also teachers who have the 'ability to get into the autistic mindset intuitively', there are others whose approach is 'confrontational'.

Larkey agrees. She asks educators to put themselves in a child's shoes. 'Imagine what it's like to walk into your classroom,' she says. What does the classroom look like? How do the children communicate? Do all the kids know each other, or are any of them trying to seek out friends? Put yourself in the shoes of every child who walks through your classroom door.

Emily Hammond, who created the popular online resource NeuroWild, says the power of an adult in the school setting cannot be underestimated. She says that too often, when a 'breakdown' occurs in class, 'the autistic kid gets singled out' and labelled as naughty or rude by an educator. Children then go home, and that news travels with stories to their own parents about their school day. 'It comes down to people recognising the huge value of difference,' she says. 'A lot of our systems, especially education, praise conformity but we don't fit into those boxes. We do things differently. But it's not wrong. It's not problematic. It's just unfamiliar to a lot of people, and unfortunately people often perceive unfamiliarity as scary or troublesome.'

TEACHING TIPS FOR ND STUDENTS

Within a school setting the culture begins at the top, where tone is usually set. And that begs the question: What does a good school culture look like? And how might you measure it?

Some teachers are employing novel ways to make genuine and lasting differences in their classroom. When we asked teachers what strategies and techniques worked well, these examples stood out, and we hope it provides a drawer full of ideas for other educators.

- 'Let them fidget, rock, provide breaks and be flexible. Build positive relationships and be a safe person and space for them.'
- 'Use the language, "Is everything okay?" and "How can I help?"'
- 'Provide a calm tent with sensory activities and fidget toys.'
- 'Provide wobble chairs and wiggle cushions.'
- 'I've used a secret signalling system – for when they feel they need a break, or to get my attention for further explanation – using the position of their calculator on the desk.'
- 'Have "brain breaks" to release dopamine – pedals, kicking a ball, stomping stairs, making Lego – but you have to find the thing for each kid.'

- 'Allow headphones.'
- 'Give classroom jobs to keep busy while the rest of the class are having group times.'
- 'Create a job of tearing up old paper in the back of the classroom when they need a break.'
- 'I send my student on errands to deliver messages to other teachers – often in the year level above so that my student gets used to next year's classrooms. The messages are usually unimportant, but it gives my ND student a break from being at the desk.'
- 'Invisible scaffolding – we put support in place that other kids don't see or notice so that our ND child doesn't stand out – because he really, really doesn't want to stand out from the other kids.'
- 'Movement breaks. I have a set of laminated cards on a table – students can choose to take one, put the card on their own desk, then do the activity just outside the classroom.'
- 'Adopt the "Zones of regulation".' (See page 124.)
- 'Reward the effort and not the outcome.'
- 'I use my fingers when giving multi-step instructions, and always keep the instructions in the same order – wash your hands, get your lunch box, sit on the mat. One of our favourite strategies is tummy-breathing time before we have lunch. This gives their bodies a chance to slow down. And gives me an opportunity to teach them about tuning in to their bodies and their needs, and feeling their heartbeat. We started with a ninety second tummy breathing session at the start of the year and now we are at about four minutes. We

introduced lavender scented eye masks this term. They love it!'
- 'Pre-teach and provide access to texts for next term, before the holidays, so kids feel like they are a step ahead.'
- 'I talk to him about his incredible self being like a Ferrari car. And with brakes that don't always work. I remind him to put on his brakes when things go wrong (pause before reacting).'
- '[Focus on] transitioning. Especially to the new year. I always make contact early in term four and get to know the child and their parents. One girl loved koalas so I wore them on my clothes when we first met. When she [first] came into the classroom, it was set up how she would find it in term one.'

ND TEACHERS

One issue that was raised during our research, was that many teachers are ND themselves. As one parent told us: 'I have a working theory that many teachers are ND and that if we unlocked those personal diagnoses it would completely change the face of education for the better, because they would have more empathy and understanding for kids through the lens of their newfound personal understanding.'

Garnett says some schools have been rewarded by welcoming back former ND students so their current students understood more about the challenges ND children face at school. It also helped others seek a diagnosis. She admits she is also better at her job because she is autistic, despite being diagnosed as an adult. She believes strong leadership is important. 'I'm just so grateful for being autistic because of what it's given me in my life. I've got an amazing ability and lovely personality characteristics because of it. But I'm also aware that it's been a massive challenge for me, and it's caused enormous social anxiety. Without the privilege I've had, and the support I've received, I could easily be very unwell as a person.' It's a raw honest assessment that should provide hope for others, and a determination to gift all of our children the support they need to reach their full potential.

Larkey says teachers need to know there will be good and bad days. 'For me, as a first year teacher, I wish someone had said to me, "You're not going to get it perfect all the time. Just keep persisting. If you keep persisting … this will be the favourite student you've ever taught."

HOW TEACHERS CAN WORK WITH PARENTS

- The single most powerful thing a teacher can do is get to know the individual child. A conversation about Pokémon, the Matildas, chess, or Harry Potter can build a connection and get that relationship off to a positive start.
- Have a handover with the child's former teacher: find out what has worked, what were the challenges, and what might help in the year ahead.
- Allow ND children and those with school anxiety the chance to drop off their books the week before school starts. Allow them to meet their teacher and see the classroom without lots of other kids around.

- Allow a child to have a friend in their class. If they've successfully made a strong friend (and it's reciprocated) allowing those children to be together in a class the following year is important.
- Meet with the parents before the school year begins, and again in week three or four to see how the child is going.
- Send an 'All About My Child' questionnaire for the parent to fill in before the school year begins. Ask about the child's strengths, areas for support, concerns and any ideas the parents may have on how to overcome challenges.
- Some ND kids benefit from an email with a photo of you and your classroom so they know what to expect before you meet.

7. TO THE PRINCIPAL'S OFFICE

'ALEX IS THE MOST INCREDIBLE BOY,' his mother says, 'the keenest fisherman you'll ever meet. He is already well known among the local fishing community, is regularly in fishing mags, has a "job" lined up at the bait store when he turns ten, and is in talks with the local council to get a bin for his favourite jetty.' Alex's mother, Kate, knows her son will add value to the world in amazing ways. 'It's just getting through the school system which is the tricky part,' she says.

Kate told us her autistic son was clever enough to tell his teachers when he was in the 'red zone'; a non-physical place where he felt he needed help to regulate his thoughts and emotions. On one occasion, his cup was filling and despite his age, he knew it would soon overflow. Autistic children are taught this early, and many schools have adopted the Zones of Regulation – a curriculum framework organised around four coloured zones to describe feelings, energy and emotions. This helps children to understand their feelings and ask for help to regulate back to a green (happy and calm) zone.

Alex knew he was becoming angry and frustrated and was entering the red zone; the one where he felt overwhelmed. He wanted to go to the monkey bars, which was an agreed upon strategy, his mother says. By the accounts of his parents, he was ignored and his behaviour escalated, until a decision was made to evacuate the classroom. Just a reminder: Alex is seven years old. Angry and lost, he trashed the room and was immediately suspended.

Alex's story, like many others, shows how the narrative for neurodivergent children is that they are naughty, uncontrollable and unable to respect others. There is a widely held view that all ND kids are disruptive, sometimes violent, and encourage bad behaviours in class. In early 2024 a federal inquiry brought down a report, 'The issue of increasing disruption in Australian school classrooms'. While that investigation wasn't into the behaviour of ND students, for many families, it pointed a finger at them.

> 'The school is okay, but I have found it's the year teacher that makes the most impact. The years that he has had a caring, thoughtful teacher, are the years that he has excelled.'

At school, ADHD boys in particular, are labelled as naughty and disruptive, and the level of school suspensions has reached epidemic proportions, with some children we spoke to having been sent home for several days at a time. As one child said: 'I'm not a bad kid but it's hard when people don't take the time to find out why something is hard for me or explain it to me. I don't want my friends to know when something is hard, so I don't ask the teacher for help and then they think I'm wasting time or not trying.'

Students with a diagnosed disability make up less than

twenty per cent of school enrolments but receive nearly half of all school suspensions. And those leading that charge, on every bit of evidence given to us during our research, were children with an 'invisible' condition, such as autism and ADHD.

The issue is: are these kids being deliberately naughty and disrespectful or is their behaviour being misinterpreted? Are their attempts at communication not being understood, despite the big banner of inclusion hung outside our schools? And if suspension is the answer, you have to wonder what the question might be, because students – from as young as five years old – are repeatedly being suspended without any change to their 'behaviour'. These incidents are often caused by a meltdown, where a child's behaviour escalates and becomes threatening or disruptive or, in some instances, violent. In many cases, furniture is upended and other children are frightened.

Given that a suspension can last from anywhere between one day to two weeks, and because a child is only allowed to return to class gradually, this has a huge impact on their self-esteem and their parents' working lives. The impact on family life is difficult to quantify, but at the very least, it means that one parent has to take leave, or in some instances give up their job, just so they can be on standby for a child who may or may not be allowed to go to school on any one day.

Let's take the example of Alex and his mother, Kate. When Alex was allowed to return to school, on one occasion it was for only forty-five minutes a day, and he was only allowed in the garden. 'He was not allowed to go back to the classroom for three weeks and remained on reduced hours for six weeks,' Kate says. 'My husband took six weeks leave from work to facilitate this. The principal informed us that there would be an incident report, which we would receive, and that already they had discovered things that did not go to plan on their end, and areas where they could improve staff knowledge and training.'

Legal advice prevented the school providing the report to Alex's parents and they had to seek assistance to access it. It showed the school's lack of planning for an episode such as this. Following the incident Kate was full of shame and offered to pay for any damage. But that shame soon dissipated and turned to disappointment, and then anger over how Alex's suspension was dealt with. Three representatives from the school sector attended the first meeting post-incident. 'It was the first sign that [Alex] was moving from a child with a disability to a risk which had to be mitigated.'

That's just the start of Alex's story and, frighteningly, it is not isolated. Both his parents are in service professions – a teacher and a police officer – and they understand mandatory reporting processes and expectations. But they were shocked by the treatment meted out to their son. Despite clear guidelines, they say they were not invited to meetings to discuss Alex's behaviour. They were later reported to child services, because of a belief their seven-year-old could endanger his family. Child safety officers quickly closed their case. They also struggled to access NDIS help for support with intensive behaviour intervention. 'I picked myself up off the floor and appealed and tried again and we got funding,' his mother says. And then, 'we won the lottery'. Well, not really, but they found a medication combination that worked to manage their son's anxiety and impulsivity.

'We cracked a combo,' she explains. 'It was life-changing.' Alex returned to school, calm and engaged. He was reading and writing. 'He was the child we always knew he could be with the right medication and supports.' But in the classroom it made little difference. 'There was no, "new term, fresh start" mentality and, even when Alex was giving his absolute all, they still refused to increase his hours by half an hour,' Kate says.

Alex's parents have been advised to go to the Human Rights Commission and the federal court, but their energy, at least at the moment, is focused on Alex. 'My priority is genuine inclusion for my child, and every other child, while I'm at it. I understand this challenge from more than one perspective. I'm a mother and a teacher and have held leadership positions. I get that this is hard. No one sets out to make life difficult for these children and their families, but if we don't know better, we can't do better.'

'Tone at the top' is a phrase we often hear in politics, or even in the corporate world, and it is just as important in our schools. 'What changes things is when a leader in the school – the principal or deputy principal, someone with power – wants to do something about it,' says autism expert and clinical psychologist Dr Michelle Garnett. Often, she says, that might happen when their own child or someone in their family is diagnosed as neurodivergent. It switches a light on, that then carries to the school, and changes are made. This is borne out in our research. One parent told us a principal agreed to part-time schooling which had changed her child's journey: 'Later found out the principal was dyslexic.'

Surely, if Australia topped the world in education school ratings, we might believe we have an inclusive education system that works – where every child is equally valued. But we don't. So why do we think the current way we deal with classroom 'behaviour' is best practice? On the advice of every expert we spoke to, it was not. But the voice here belongs to those families who are dealing with this today and tomorrow and next week.

DETENTIONS AND SUSPENSIONS

Monique's son was suspended eight times in Prep, and then could only attend school two hours a day until he – and his parents – completed behaviour training. Monique's son would lash out at others when he saw something he didn't like. In one case, he saw a child push someone else to jump position in a queue. His sense of social justice – an attribute in many autistic children – meant he then pushed that person back. From that first suspension, Monique said, her son was watched. Other parents would say their child had been touched by Monique's son, and the school's response was an immediate suspension. He only started his first full day of school in Year 2. Monique's husband was forced to take a redundancy.

'[Our son] understood he was being suspended and that meant he couldn't go to school. In terms of confidence, he internalised it. He started to think he was being watched by everyone. No one was watching what the other boys were doing.' A stigma set in: he was a troublemaker. Monique describes a neurodivergent child – not all, but many – as a spray of water coming out of a shower head. It might spray in a different direction to all the others, but 'with the use of strategies … it just all comes together'.

That's not the case for Eloise, who had twenty-eight suspensions during Year 7. 'She had severe separation anxiety and would use her phone to communicate with me throughout the day,' her mother told us. This strategy had been agreed upon at meetings with the school, but some teachers would not allow it. Eloise would then be suspended, return to school, only to be suspended again. On multiple occasions she was sent home to 'cool off'. 'She was sent home over forty times last year alone,' her mother says. 'Every school day I would have multiple phone calls from many of her teachers, student services and the principal. At no point did they realise it wasn't working in suspending her.'

Garnett says we should be 'diagnosing the system' rather than punishing children. 'Talk about rigid! Who's got the problem here?' she asks. 'There must be open-mindedness. The schools must be willing to learn. They need flexibility.' She goes on to emphasise that as well as understanding the child and parents' point of view, we need compassion for the teachers, too. 'I honestly feel so sorry for teachers at the moment. I used to want to be a teacher. They're just so under-resourced and under-educated for the complex difficulties they need to deal with.'

Educator and autism advocate Sue Larkey agrees: 'The child's not coping because the system's not coping. It's just a symptom of a system, isn't it? Sending a child to the office doesn't give them the tools to emotionally regulate. The higher your anxiety, the less you can regulate. What is the point of sending a child to the office? What are they learning? Nothing. If a child's been suspended twenty-eight times, I'd ask the principal: What's the educational outcome? What is the child learning from being at home?'

Linda Graham, a QUT professor and director of The Centre for Inclusive Education agrees. 'But it doesn't surprise me all that much,' she says. 'I wish I could say that it did.'

Graham has worked in this area for years and says it's an issue playing out in schools across the country. In one case, she was told of a thirteen-year-old boy who had successive suspensions that stretched for months. 'He'd been out of school for eighteen months, travelling around in his dad's truck, because he had nowhere else to go.'

Another mother shared the impact that her son's suspensions were having on their family. 'As a single mother who has never had any family support for fifteen years and worked full-time to support my children and pay my mortgage, I was suicidal and on the verge of a nervous breakdown. The school was calling me to pick him up before I had even gotten to work in the morning. He has missed out on months of school due to suspensions and I've been asked to keep him home to give him a rest.' The pressure on her was enormous: she couldn't afford, financially, to leave her job, but her child was suffering and she was desperate to walk beside him. 'I couldn't do anything,' she said.

Suspension usually follows detention, although a visit to the principal's office or calling parents to pick up their child were also common disciplinary measures. 'Suspended once, but in the same year he had sixty absences or early finishes due to calls to pick him up early or needing rest days,' says one parent. Another says, 'My daughter was never suspended, just several phone calls home to come and get her. I was always on edge, waiting for them to call.'

Larkey says there are often 'subtle signs' in the lead-up to most meltdowns. 'A little bit of redness in the face, a child whose hair is a bit ruffled – these are all signs that child needs a break.' Outbursts don't just come 'from nowhere'. 'One day, the child probably could handle someone knocking everything off their desk. It depends where they're at.' She likens it to a driver in traffic. In a good mood, it might not perturb us. 'The next day someone cuts you off and you get really angry – it's no different for our children.'

We need to put ourselves in their shoes, Larkey says. 'Everyone has good and bad days, but what we're doing is sending this kid home on a bad day, which isn't changing anything. We need to be proactive, not reactive. I don't think any reactive strategies have been proven, clinically, to work. Show me the research that says suspension and expulsion actually fixes misbehaviour – I haven't seen it.' And yet, it appears to be the standard course of action in schools' behaviour management.

Many of the families we spoke to confirmed that suspensions were not having the desired effect on their children. 'Four suspensions so far this year. Just finished a ten-day one today. Suspension does not change his response but does lower his self-esteem, increase his anxiety and damage his reputation.' Another noted: 'In Year 1, my daughter was told not to return for the last two weeks of term four, as they couldn't handle her. She thought she had been "fired" from school.' As another mother observed: 'The irony is that these suspensions and school changes have been very damaging, resulting in social and academic disconnection and leading to greater likelihood of future incidents.'

The solution to this is tricky – but what is clear is that suspensions are not working, and the role of the school here needs to be put in the headlights. Principals and senior educators need to consider all of their students – including and perhaps especially their ND students – and ensure that staff are not only aware of what behavioural issues to look out for but are given strategies to deal with them so that all students can benefit. There seem to be no best-practice policies in operation broadly across the education system, with schools adopting and implementing their own strategies – and almost always without consultation with the ND community who are most affected by them. 'The school wants the children to sign contracts that they won't do anything wrong, but the school won't put in writing what they will do to deter bad behaviour in unstructured play,' one parent observed.

The difference in how schools dealt with bullying and other behavioural issues stood out in our research: 'When my child was at his old school, he was regularly labelled the naughty kid and would be "orange carded" for absent-minded misdemeanours.' The new school has strong routines and structures in place, movement breaks and a high ratio of teachers to students. 'He has not had a single misdemeanour incident and is seen as well behaved, caring and conscientious.' At this school, teachers had all attended courses for students who might have individual needs.

> 'My son was excluded from incursions, excursions, camps and sports at his old school. He had multiple suspensions. Since moving to a new school, he's joined in every activity and is considered a school leader.'

Another parent said: 'We picked an amazing school [that] truly look at what is behind the behaviour and address the cause.' There were many other positive experiences where schools were proactively dealing with ND kids. 'The principal said to me at our initial interview, "He is exactly who he is meant to be. Our job as educators is to adapt the classroom so he can be the best he can be at school."'

Autism and neurodiversity support specialist Kristy Forbes says that punitive measures shouldn't be used against ND children – but many parents don't have other school options. Forbes said it was a 'privilege' to be able to homeschool a child. 'We don't have the type of system that would support families to be able to bring their children home.' She says a neuro-normative world is focused on academia, success, productivity and achievement, and parents don't have access to those stories of people who didn't make it through the school system, but later completed multiple university degrees or reached similar levels of 'success' via another route. This is a message for all families: an ATAR is not the only path to higher educationn but this can be hard to believe as the push by some schools to lead achievement league tables of Year 12 academic merit is often prioritised over other avenues to success.

Larkey says one of the biggest issues with the education system is that schools' claims of being inclusive run counter to the suspension, attendance and homeschooling rates we are seeing. She says inclusivity could be judged in other ways. For example, how many social gatherings is a child invited to attend? Does the principal ever receive emails from parents asking that their child not mix with another child? 'If we're inclusive, why would parents think it's okay to send an email like that?' Larkey says children see on social media they have been excluded and she asks parents this question: 'Would you want to turn up at your next book club if all your friends went away on the weekend and you weren't invited?'

Professor Linda Graham says schools also know what they are doing is not working, 'but they don't know what else to do'. She says a child is often suspended because 'we sacrifice the rights of one' to grant the rights of most others. But other reasons exist, with principals saying it 'gave the teacher a break'. Sometimes teachers 'gang up against the principal … they want the child out. I've been in schools where there's been kids excluded, where the principal does not want to do it.' The principal might know the child wasn't intentionally disruptive but is forced to act 'when a significant number of staff get together and say, "We don't feel safe."' She says teachers are feeling 'under siege a lot of the time' and the rising number of suspensions also spoke to a 'stressed profession'.

WHEN BULLIED CHILDREN FIGHT BACK

In many of the stories we were told, a neurodivergent child lashed out after they were provoked. Sometimes the provocation was overt – knocking their sandwich out of their hand or bumping into them, flicking their neck as they walk past or waiting until the teacher's back was turned before reaching over and messing up their coloured pencils. Teasing. Tormenting. Smirking.

As one parent told us: 'Another child was lining up for class and told my son to hold a vape, and being naive and happy that this child was talking to him, my son took the vape and held it for the child – which then led to a suspension.'

Our research revealed that many ND children were frequently being bullied, and the outcome of these destructive peer interactions was varied. For example, one mother told us that her son was bullied for twelve months, with peers regularly taking his bag, shoes and phone from him. He retaliated and was later suspended. What was the impact? 'He learnt not to defend himself or retaliate, ever.' So, the bullying and sense of isolation only increased.

Graham says the impact of a suspension is so damaging that it should not be considered at any point. 'There's a lot of rhetoric around it being the option of last resort. Well, I call BS on that. It is not the option of last resort. To be honest, I think it has to be taken off the table as an option.'

A point that shone out across states and education sectors is that the tone is set from the top and, as we highlighted earlier, one teacher can make a world of difference. As one parent explained: '[He] had gotten beaten up by an older child. The teacher emailed me explaining what had happened. I ran to him to see how he was and asked him questions. He didn't really explain what had happened just said it was true. My heart broke for him. Like he just accepted it. I felt disconnected even more. I emailed the principal explaining the situation. They suspended the boy [who assaulted him].'

In many cases, parents nominated school avoidance as the impact of being in trouble at school. In some cases, children had not been to school for two-and-a-half years. And for many, it becomes a vicious circle. A child can miss days and weeks of learning, thereby putting them behind where they might have otherwise been, and in a position where they are forced to play catch-up repeatedly, which can then create a new cycle of anxiety.

PERFECT AT SCHOOL, MELTDOWNS AT HOME

Some ND children will mask or camouflage during the day, copying other children in the hope of fitting in with their peers. 'My daughter is extremely good at masking and so she tends to be able to "hold it together" at school but then has massive meltdowns either before or after school.' They will work to ensure they are never singled out as being naughty or badly behaved. 'Rules are very important to my girl and she will always follow them, also she is a high-masking autistic and tends to shut down rather than meltdown, so she rarely gets in trouble.'

Many ND children are able to regulate themselves and not be the focus of complaints about their behaviour. As one parent identified: 'That is only one profile. The other danger is the introvert, who flies under the radar, tries not to rock the boat, wants to do the class work, but can't access it the way it is presented, or can't respond fluently in the format demanded. They seek teacher help, but then the teacher says, "I already explained that!" So, they sit there and feel demoralised, disenfranchised, stupid and afraid to speak up again. They are at risk of learning failure, anxiety, depression and self-harm. They are the quiet ones who carry the blackness and hopelessness of the system inside them, and incorrectly attribute the failure of the system as their own failure. Who is helping the ones quietly dying inside the system, not wanting to attract further teacher disdain?'

Other parents had similar stories: 'My daughter is scared of being in trouble so will just go quiet. She is likely to be the one to go unnoticed and learn nothing due to that [rather] than being the disruptive child.'

By trying to stay out of trouble, some kids end up isolating themselves further in their peer group. 'I have an angel here who would be mortified to get in trouble. He's never been in trouble once and his report card says he "has a keen sense of justice" … so he's more of a dobber, if anything.'

Kids who camouflage all day often experience meltdowns when they get home. As one parent told us: 'Our daughter is the "perfect student" and at home it all falls apart.' And: 'My kids are maskers. So, they are angels at school and explode at home. Teachers often think I'm crazy and find it hard to imagine.'

Overwhelmingly, those who mask at school cave in once they walk through the front door of their home. 'They save it all up for at home,' one parent said. And that means nightly emotional outbursts.

CANARIES IN THE COAL MINE

Graham says problems within the education system are multifaceted, and one approach to solving them is to 'start seeing these kids as the canaries in the coal mine'. She explains her analogy: 'Many years ago, coal miners used to take canaries in cages down into the coal mines because the canaries were a very good indicator of when oxygen was running out. "Canary in the coal mine" is basically an expression about the stress in a system'; they are like a beacon going to raise the alarm that 'all is not right'.

In our survey, teachers repeatedly raised the work of American psychologist Dr Ross Greene. On the faculty at Harvard Medical School for more than two decades, Greene is now founding director of the non-profit Lives in the Balance, which provides resources around the Collaborative and Proactive Solutions (CPS) model for classrooms.

The CPS model is different from others in several ways. Firstly, Greene tells us, it focuses less on a child's behaviour, and more on what might be 'causing that behaviour'. Secondly, it engages the child as part of the problem-solving process; the key stakeholder in how it will be fixed. And finally, it aims to be proactive, rather than in response to an incident. He says the approach is not limited to any diagnosis: a child might be autistic, have ADHD, ODD, or a host of other conditions. 'All the diagnosis does is summarise the behaviour that kid is exhibiting,' he says.

In short, the CPS model is based on the understanding that challenging behaviour happens when expectations placed on a child are bigger than their capacity to respond. Some children have more skills than others to adapt – so the model focuses less on their behaviour and more on how they are communicating their difficulty in meeting what they are required to do. Teachers need to know 'what's happening early and what's happening late' with a child. 'What's happening early is the expectation the kid is having difficulty meeting. What's happening after is the way the kid is communicating they're having difficulty meeting that expectation – which is their concerning behaviour,' he says. 'So, number one, I want to make sure that teachers are not focused on making a list of those concerning behaviours and trying to come up with innovative ways to modify those behaviours. There are no innovative ways to modify behaviours, it's been the same for fifty years – it's either a reward, or it's a punishment in one form or another. I don't think there's a lot of innovation there.' The teacher, he says, instead needs to focus on the child's 'unmet expectations' or 'unsolved problems'. Irrespective of if the teacher is new or established, changing focus is crucial. 'Are you focused on the right thing?'

Unsolved problems can be identified using a tool called the *Assessment of Skills and Unsolved Problems* (ASUP). The ASUP is an online resource provided by Lives in the Balance and was designed as a discussion guide, rather than as a checklist or rating scale, to assist with identifying lagging skills and proactively addressing problems.

Once the problems are understood, they become 'highly predictable' and solvable in a proactive way. Greene argues this is a more effective strategy as it means outbursts are less likely, and so is the need to employ de-escalation techniques. When asked if this might be difficult for a teacher who might have thirty children in a class, Greene's response is instant. 'They'll have thirty children in the class whether they're doing the right thing or the wrong thing,' he says.

When asked if the schools are doing enough to include kids

with diverse needs in the classroom, Greene says: 'Increasingly, yes. Are we teaching our educators how to deal with all that diversity as effectively as possible? I would say the answer is still no.'

So, what advice would Greene offer teachers who may be walking into a class today, where several students are ND – some diagnosed, others not?

'If a kid is struggling to meet your expectations, use the ASUP instrument. Figure out who you've got in your classroom and start solving problems collaboratively and proactively. And I say that, regardless of whether the child is ND or NT.'

Teachers, Greene says, are aware that old models of behaviour management are not working. 'They are becoming increasingly aware of the price we all pay for getting it wrong. It's not just the kids who pay the price, not just their parents who pay the price – their classmates pay the price when they see a kid who continues to be treated in a way that isn't working.'

Greene believes that the world is opening up to individual differences. 'The ND community has been leading the way on that.' They are using their voice to ensure people understand neurodivergence better, and in the process are educating everyone. 'I'm optimistic because I think this is the direction we're heading in.'

8. FROM THE TEACHER'S DESK

IN ANY DISCUSSION ABOUT TEACHING in classrooms, and how neurodivergent students fit in, it's important to hear the voices of teachers, who often feel undervalued and easily maligned. Our educational respondents were drawn from public, private and independent schools. Some of them were junior staff, having recently graduated from university, with long careers in front of them. Others have taught two generations of students. Some are focused on young children in primary school, while others are secondary teachers, who are preparing students for those final tests before they head off into their own futures – whether that involves further learning or joining the workforce.

Before we can make improvements toward an inclusive education system, we have to take a step inside those classroom doors where teachers stand in front of our children. This is important, because while we have discussed the needs of ND students and their families, educators are crucial in delivering results. Yet, how much thought is given to those professionals who we charge with filling our children's minds with curiosity and a willingness to learn?

Karen has a student in Year 4 who is smart, funny, intelligent, unique, kind, caring and neurodivergent. 'Unfortunately, her parents think all her stimming, meltdowns and anxiety attacks are just to get their attention and they refuse to get her diagnosed. She can scream so loud we have to evacuate the building. She picks her skin all day and has sores over her arms and legs.' Karen says this young girl has never seen a therapist and doesn't understand what is happening to her. 'She holds a special place in my heart, and I really wish I could do more to help her.'

Karen is one teacher out of 600 who answered our questions about ND children in their classrooms. She's not alone in wondering how she might help the students sitting in front of her. Another teacher talks about a Year 11 student who has ADHD and dyslexia, who is behind his peers academically. 'This young man will not receive help, the stigma attached to receiving support is so negative in his eyes, he does not want to receive any extra assistance. He also explains that he doesn't like to "pull the dyslexia card".'

A third teacher wants to talk about Sally: 'She flies under the radar. She seems quiet. She uses every inch of energy she has to fit in. She mimics others, she has already learnt that, at seven years old, everything she does is wrong, so the best strategy is to copy others – that way she'll blend in and she won't get in trouble.' A fourth teacher talks about her 'amazing talented drawer, who is incredibly smart, (and) desperately wants friends'. She is kind to others 'even when they are not'.

'These wonderful students are why we get up and do what we do each day,' another teacher says. Yet another singles out her highly intelligent Year 1 student who has limited vocabulary and social understanding. 'Children think she is a baby until she can open nearly any book and read it,' she says.

Read on, and you will find delightful examples of how teachers have learnt from the children in front of them. But firstly, it's worth highlighting the complexity that teachers are facing, where educators are navigating large class sizes, filled with students with widely different learning abilities and different neurodivergencies.

In previous chapters, we've given the voice to parents and children, but teachers are instrumental here, too, and this chapter explores how they see their job teaching a class of individual learners. They told us that some parents become accusatory in a bid to advocate for their ND child. Others do not want their child to undergo a diagnosis because of the fear they believe a label will deliver. Funding is patchy, resources are limited and many teachers admit their own knowledge of diversity is lacking, having only limited education at university to deliver personalised lessons to suit ND students. They all recognised there were few professional development opportunities they could access.

TEACHERS ON THE FRONTLINE

There are a wide variety of students who fall under the ND umbrella, including those who have been officially diagnosed and those who show numerous traits. Teachers told us that the number of students in their classes they believe are ND is much higher than the public discussion enveloping it. A common belief in the teaching profession is that up to forty per cent of some classes show ND characteristics, but only as few as five per cent are diagnosed, with many skilled at masking. Some teachers were specific: 'Forty-eight per cent in my class have a diagnosis or are in the process of getting a diagnosis.' Others, who acted as tutors, said as many as seventy per cent of their students were

ND. Numbers were reported as higher in some demographics: 'I'm in a low socioeconomic area – high trauma. I would say between sixty and seventy per cent are neurodivergent, not all are diagnosed though.'

This raises again the inequity between those families who can afford to go down the path of diagnosis – visiting therapists, psychologists and specialists – and those who cannot. These high estimates are difficult to comprehend compared with those routinely quoted for autism (between one in thirty and one in seventy people) and ADHD (about one in twenty). Teachers believe their estimates are more accurate, however, based on a number of factors that are not considered in other data – the fact that so many girls mask their condition; the number of children who are undiagnosed despite experiencing obvious challenges; as well as those waiting in queues for a diagnosis. Much of that is not in reported data. As one teacher told us: 'I have a countless list of paediatrician surveys to fill in for children every year. More than ever before.'

A primary school deputy principal said educating a broad spectrum of students has become more complex over the past two decades. 'We have a lot of students diagnosed/verified, but the number of students we support with imputed ND is high because parents don't want a label on their child,' she said. In other cases, a family has a diagnosis but does not want to share it with the school. Dozens of teachers also pointed to the fact that particular subjects in high school might carry a greater proportion of ND students. For example, enrolment in Game Design and Development in senior school could be as high as fifty per cent, while in younger years, compulsory subjects carried a ratio of one in ten. 'It varies depending on the class,' another high-school teacher said. 'My ability to identify ND kids (verified and non-verified) has changed dramatically since having ND kids myself.'

The power of a teacher has been outlined in Chapter 6, but how teachers see their own ability to educate ND children is particularly illuminating. Some teachers have been granted regular professional development in autism and ADHD. Others who identified as ND were filled to the brim with knowledge. Those who had a ND child also had sought information and skills to help navigate the path at home. They were then able to apply that in the classroom, and found it was a game-changer. Others have undertaken postgraduate training, including Master's degrees, to explore areas of neurodivergence and ensure they are confident in front of their class. Many have done this at their own expense.

Some teachers have received information during sporadic professional development (PD) days, including accessing extra resources, participating in online workshops and visiting experts. A lot of teachers reported their experience has been acquired in response to what they call 'behaviour management' on the job. 'The majority of what I know has come from working with ND children, talking to their parents, speaking to special education teachers. I also learnt a lot when my own husband sought a ADHD diagnosis as an adult,' one teacher told us.

But, the majority of teachers who responded to our survey did not have any personal experience with neurodivergence, and their education in the area was negligible. As one teacher told us: 'I attended PD with an organisation in 2016 but haven't had any further PD since.' Another experienced teacher said: 'Very little over thirty years of teaching.' Another admitted 'Nowhere near enough. An occasional fifteen-minute chat during a staff meeting.'

Mostly, teachers had sought out information themselves, prompted by a student they were teaching. In almost all cases this education – whether it be further reading, podcasts or online courses and webinars – was done at the teacher's own expense and in their own time.

> *'It is about knowing your student, their triggers, their strengths and adjustments that work for them.'*

Dr Ross Greene's CPS approach had been explained in some schools, and some had participated in Sue Larkey's workshops. Other teachers raised the work of Professor Tony Attwood, while others sought valuable resources from Yellow Ladybugs, SPELD Queensland, Amaze, Autism Queensland and a host of other autism, ADHD and PDA experts. Many teachers believed training and resources around autism were easier to find than other ND conditions. 'Any training offered has generally had to be in my own time and volition and I've had to hunt it down,' one teacher told us. Another pleaded for universities to teach education students about 'early child brain development, generational poverty, trauma and how these things impact on brain development'.

CHALLENGES IN THE CLASSROOM

Undoubtedly, across the board, teachers are attempting to understand each of their students, a task made more difficult when a child is undiagnosed and parents are unwilling to entertain an investigation. The stories that follow are told by teachers and show how a single child can throw up significant challenges to time-poor teachers, who must meet curriculum benchmarks, undertake more administrative tasks than ever before, and teach another twenty-five students; many of whom also carry challenges.

- 'Master J is ADHD. He is very bright but struggles to settle and stay focused. Medication was helping him immensely and because he was focused his grades began to pick up. Not long after we noticed a decline in attention and focus. After contacting the parent I was told he had been removed from medication. It has been a struggle for the remainder of the year for him without medication.'
- 'Gosh, where to start? There is one who really struggles with appropriate timing for jokes and can't tell when they need to respond to the demands of the classroom in a serious manner. Due to this, and his social challenges, he really struggles to be accepted and it is difficult to make friends.'
- '[I have a student] who often screams, throws tantrums, leaves class and barely completes any schoolwork. No social skills, unable to share or take turns. No diagnosis and no funding for this student.'
- '[She] does not like eye contact, arms flap when excited, not diagnosed.'
- 'I have a Year 1 student who is diagnosed ADHD, unmedicated. Very violent, beginning to be more so towards other students and staff. Mum acts supportive and appears on top of everything but excuses his behaviour and tries to blame the school. Mum has a lot of shame attached to his behaviour.'
- '[He] finds the whole environment of pre-primary overwhelming – the noise, the other children, the space,

the fact that it's not home. He is mostly nonverbal, will echo things said to him by others but doesn't use language to convey needs. Still in nappies at four-and-a-half years old. The school in this case has provided funds for an education assistant. Without this, we have no way of providing the downtime M needs while still providing supervision to other students.'

- 'She bites, scratches, screams, picks her nose and wipes it on students; puts her fingers inside her underpants and then puts them in her mouth. Classroom frequently evacuated for safety reasons.'
- 'I have one student who is particularly challenging across all areas, with staff often complaining of aggressive, explosive behaviour. She has been suspended on multiple occasions. I see so much of my own ND child in her, a kid who just wants to feel that she is accepted for who she is and shown unconditional safety and support, understanding and care. Sadly, she has been labelled from the get-go and rather than look beyond the behaviour to other factors that are contributing to her challenges, many in the school see only the behaviour. What I see is a tormented, misunderstood, lonely and fearful child who just wants to know that someone cares. Her cries for help get louder and her behaviours more concerning – self-harm, aggression and violence, property damage – yet she and I are not listened to, rather she is plastered with a label that is now so set that she will never escape it. My heart breaks for her every single day.'
- 'I had a student in Year 8. I knew almost immediately he had ADHD. He was a lovely student but could not concentrate. His mum was so lovely and after multiple

calls asked point blank whether she should get him tested, I said yes. After many months he was diagnosed, he was prescribed medication and suddenly started passing subjects. Here is the thing: I kept thinking, why wasn't this kid recognised earlier? Was he labelled as naughty? Age thirteen, in my opinion, is far too late. He was moved to my class because his other teacher "couldn't handle him", which just makes me so sad.'

- 'This child is seven. He can't sit still, is easily irritated, and will lash out at students or teachers. [His] violence can be so bad we often evacuate our classroom for safety. [He] has completely trashed the classroom and the principal's office several times – this includes tearing things off walls, throwing furniture and items, emptying cupboards. He is not toilet trained and has poor social skills. He frequently swears and makes inappropriate noises.'
- 'I had a child who would only speak to me if I called him Mister Kangaroo. Once settled, he appeared like a typical little boy, his neurodiversity will become more apparent as he grows up. He is such a truly delightful child.'
- 'He is the best! He is creative, he is loyal, and he is so funny. He can learn by osmosis. We are in fits of laughter daily. And yes, some days are harder than others. Some days he will be defiant, some days he will run out of the room without telling me where he is going. Some days he is very heightened and needs reminders about the time and place of "loud noises". I always say to my class, "He isn't deciding to wake up and do the wrong behaviour, his brain works differently to yours and mine, just like all our brains are different." The kids genuinely celebrate his

success, and even sometimes remind him, gently, that it is time for a sensory break, or even better, ask him to help them with their drawings.'
- 'I have a student who I suspect has ADHD, ODD or PDA and anxiety and autism. He is currently not being very successful in my class. I have tried so many strategies that have helped other ND students, but it has been such a struggle to engage him. His family have not taken him to a paediatrician or school-based psychologist even though we have made repeated requests. He is about to go to high school, and I am very concerned.'

THRIVING IN THE CLASSROOM

So, how do teachers see ND students positively impacting their class? Overwhelmingly, teachers believe their ND students have fostered a culture of kindness and inclusion. As one teacher observed, although it isn't always easy dealing with difference, it can be very rewarding: 'I had a child who *wouldn't* stop talking. He would fill any tiny bit of silence with a comment or question. Questions that would derail the lessons every time, and encourage other students to chime in. For example: How high is the sky? Who invented school? Did you know that … His curiosity, coupled with ADHD and autism, really were the perfect combination. But it was so exhausting! It had been a particularly rough year with this kid, on top of a bunch of other challenging behaviours in the classroom, and I was unashamedly counting down the days until the term four break. One day, while I was talking to a child about their behaviour, this child comes up to me and says, "Miss, did you know that God said to love others before yourself?"

'I'm not religious, so I kind of gave an answer like, "Oh, well, there you go."

'The kid stopped in his tracks, looked me in the eye and said, "Yep, and I love you," then gave me the biggest hug. Then other students started saying it and joining in with the hug. By the end, it had morphed into this big group hug with me stuck in the centre and kids telling me they loved me (even the child I was talking to about their difficult behaviour).

'This kid, as exhausting as he was, brought excitement to the classroom. The class grew to love his constant questioning and loved debating his very philosophical questions.'

Many teachers told us how their ND students have opened up new interests for other children, created empathy and new avenues to connect. They have raised out of the box ideas, and boosted class creativity. Different perspectives and humour abound. As one teacher said: 'I had a neurodivergent student who I called my human calculator. He was amazing in calculating things quicker than I could. His quick recall really spurred on my students into learning their number facts so they could keep up with him!' Another told us: 'One started a cartoon drawing club! Kids came once a week to make graphic novels and write funny books. Another student connected with the class by sharing their love of *The 13-Storey Treehouse*, and had everyone reading the books and designing their own treehouses.'

Among the many positive stories we heard about the value of difference, it was the unique strengths of character that shone through, as one teacher noted: 'They often think more deeply, rather than accept what is being taught, and when confident [they] ask great questions.' Another agreed: 'The other students learn what it's like to be accepting and non-judgemental — that everyone's brains work differently, and we should appreciate people for who they are, not who we want them to be.' And yet rarely do these positive attributes become part of the national discussion around neurodiversity; we don't talk enough about the attributes ND children teach their classmates.

> **HOW TO BUILD A POSITIVE RELATIONSHIP WITH YOUR CHILD'S TEACHER**
>
> Former English teacher, and founder of online learning platform Scholarly, Jane Sullivan, recommends the following advice for parents when it comes to building a strong relationship with your child's teachers.
>
> 1. **HELP TEACHERS GET TO KNOW YOUR CHILD:** Your child might be one of more than a hundred students a teacher sees each week. That means no teacher will know your child as well as you. If they are struggling, reach out and let their teacher know. Be sure to contact the school with any relevant information or diagnosis that may help in understanding your child's specific needs. Remember, schools are constantly changing – new staff, new timetables, new curriculum. By being an advocate for your child, you'll ensure that the lines of communication are kept open.
> 2. **BE ON THE SAME TEAM:** The teacher is not the enemy. Students can sometimes come home with stories about what happened in class, painting the teacher in an unflattering light. An 'us against them' dynamic doesn't benefit either side. Remember that teachers are there

to help students learn and achieve their personal best. Don't talk negatively about them in front of your child. Treating your child's teacher with respect, and seeing yourself as being on the same team, sends a powerful message to your child that there is a network of support for them – at home and at school.

3. **BE RESPECTFUL OF THE TEACHER'S TIME:** Good communication is paramount in schools. And an effective teacher is a present, engaged teacher. We don't want our teachers checking emails or responding to messages mid-lesson. That means we need to be patient. Allow a reasonable time for your child's teacher to respond to your email or phone call.

4. **BE CURIOUS ABOUT YOUR CHILD'S LEARNING:** Every parent can relate to the blank stare and mumbled, 'I dunno,' that meets their daily enquiry, 'What did you learn at school today?' Perhaps a better way to understand what your child is learning is to read the classroom newsletters, download their work programs or assessment schedules and ask specific questions, such as: 'I can see you're studying *Hamlet* this term, what do you think of Shakespeare?' By actively engaging with what they are learning, you will be able to ask the teacher for more specific guidance or support. Being curious is a great way to stay connected with your child, and their teacher.

5. **GET INVOLVED WITH THE SCHOOL:** Schools love parental involvement. When parents volunteer at sports carnivals or participate in fundraising activities or visit the classroom to help with literacy programs, students begin to see school and home as a partnership.

> 6. **SHOW YOUR APPRECIATION:** Most teachers enter the profession because they have a passion for working with young people and want to help them succeed. They work hard at school, and at home, to create engaging, thoughtful lessons. Consider taking the time to say, 'thank you'. Showing appreciation is a wonderful way to build a great relationship with your child's teacher.

WHAT TEACHERS WANT PARENTS TO KNOW

Despite recognising the many advantages, teachers also admitted to feeling ill-equipped to deal with such wide diversity in their classes. The disruption to other students – even minor – could have a ripple effect, including complaints by other parents. Teachers told us that the amount of communication parents expect can be exhausting, in terms of both time and difficulty, with many parents arguing that 'every child has a right to learn and that includes non-ND students, too'.

While most parents correspond respectfully, some do not, and most teachers have examples of parents who have been rude, judgemental and aggressive. 'Some are very challenging, writing long emails, or turning up during the day to speak to a teacher while we're teaching. It is turning teachers away from the profession in droves,' one teacher said. Another said she wanted parents to advocate for their children but 'when they're against you, it's soul-destroying'.

Class sizes, and not knowing how to support a child when their family is not engaged with support services or will not seek a diagnosis, is a growing problem. High-school teachers admit that knowing each ND child in secondary school, where they skip in and out of classes based on subject timetables, makes it almost impossible to understand their journey enough to always add value.

> *'There is not enough planning time for teachers to genuinely differentiate in the way that suits each child. Not every ADHD child is the same and their needs are different. Same for autism. Blanket alterations don't work.'*

Creating awareness throughout the school community is a big stumbling block to change, as one teacher noted: 'The biggest issue is when we have violent ND students in mainstream classes. Too many people think it's just bad behaviour, but it is so complex. Getting ND children to find a different behaviour to express themselves is hard but doable with proper engagement. But having parents concerned for the safety of their own child is justified, too.'

Another said: '[I'm] busting my ass to help the family trust the system and the student to love learning, when I know that it's likely that the same system will let them down repeatedly over coming years. The funding is awful, understanding of ND is awful and teacher burnout is awful. Something has got to give.' Or, as another noted; 'A teacher might turn their classroom upside down in a bid to make it compatible for learning, but outside those doors, at lunchtime, those same sensory adjustments are forgotten.'

These examples, in the words of teachers, loop back to the breadth of the problem. In any class, the mix of challenges is high: from developmental delays to non-English speaking students and refugees, others who are disengaged or whose reading level is two years behind their peers, children who have suffered trauma or have significant health issues, including allergies. 'We have to simply do our best with what we have. More people on the ground inevitably helps, but there is also a lot of extra planning, programming and preparation that I have to do in order to utilise those people in a supportive and effective way.'

Other issues raised by teachers included a lack of support, which means teachers feel they are alone in dealing with classes, evacuations prompted by classroom incidents, and having to 'conform' to traditional teaching settings. 'Unreasonable' advocacy by parents, and the broader community value put on the role of educators also influenced morale. 'As primary-school teachers, we read many reports from many "experts" who have assessed, treated, seen the ND child. We are expected to take on board their recommendations – experts who see this child maybe once, or once a month, or once a year. However, in the big round-table conference, my experience as the classroom teacher, who sees the child for five or six hours a day, is rarely seen as an expert on the child. I'm "just the teacher". It's infuriating when my thoughts, opinions and ideas are ignored, dismissed and seen as not valid as I'm not the "expert".'

And that might be the nub of the matter. When society pays educators poorly, and doesn't recognise the breadth of their role, it undervalues their place in the education of our children. This isn't about money; few teachers sign up for the pay packet. But it's about respecting the role they play. Too often their voice is muted in the debate around how our children are educated. And in the neurodivergent space, we cannot afford that. Any of us.

DEAR PARENTS,

So, what do teachers want parents to know? The answers that teachers provided to us highlight the value of communication with an emphasis on a triangular model of support — between parent, school and child — for best outcomes.

- 'Firstly, you are doing a terrific job. Secondly, I wish I had more time and resources to give your child. Lastly, I spend hours thinking about your child. I understand that behaviour is a form of communication. Let's work together to find out what your child is trying to tell us.'
- 'I care about your child. I want them to learn. But sometimes learning how to be in a classroom and interact with their peers *is learning*.'
- 'Let's pursue diagnosis to work out how we can best support your child to thrive.'
- 'There is no shame in seeking a diagnosis.'
- 'A label isn't a bad thing. It means understanding, it means targeted strategies and support, it means access to learning and specialists.'
- 'ND isn't a problem. It should be celebrated.'
- 'Your child is not flawed! They just have a different operating system.'
- 'I am doing the best I can. Your child has complex needs but so do six others in the class. I cannot meet all of their needs all of the time.'
- 'Sometimes, your child is not who they are at home and make choices that inhibit their learning. Or they are not engaging with the strategies we employ to help them.

Sometimes, your lovely ND child uses their headphone exemption/modification to watch TV shows in my class instead of to just block noise. Sometimes we cannot beat the pull of their friends and asking us to do more when your child won't meet us halfway is unfair and won't help. Approach teachers with curiosity and kindness, and we will work so bloody hard for you and your kid.'
- 'Your child is not broken, they are unique. They are why this world is so special. Don't worry about what others think or say; let go of your own preconceived ideas and embrace them for who they are. Also be strong. You are your child's biggest advocate.'
- 'We cry over our students. We fight for them. We lose sleep over them. We wish we could do and give everything your child might need, but sometimes we don't have the capacity or resources, and sometimes your child's needs might directly affect others negatively.'
- 'My ND students are my greatest teachers and make my heart sing.'
- 'Stop inventing symptoms to gain an upper hand – the amount of bullying and badgering that parents do to get what they want is ridiculous!'
- 'We need to work as a team. You know them at home, I know them at school. Communication is critical.'

PART III: SPREADING YOUR WINGS

9. JOIN A CLUB AND GET THE GOLDEN TICKET

If Pokémon is your thing, Frank Brown has what you need. Brown is the general manager of CTC Games, a Pokémon mecca housed in an industrial area about fifteen kilometres south-west of Brisbane's city centre. From the outside, the building doesn't look flash, but step inside and a Pokémon magic turns frowns into smiles. Brown has created a safe place for neurodivergent tweens and teens to socialise with like-minded people. It's a reminder that support networks are slowly becoming more available. 'I see myself at their ages in terms of social interactions and I feel envious to a point,' Brown says. 'I want to make sure these kids, who might have the support now, continue to get it from those of us who might not have had it.' CTC Games is not just for teens; kids as young as five are joined by their grandparents in their seventies and eighties, who come to learn how to play Pokémon.

Pokémon (short for Pocket Monsters) is a game of creatures who can be caught and trained by 'trainers', or humans. The Pokémon franchise includes cartoons, video games and all sorts of merchandise. Almost every school has children obsessed with collecting the cards, watching the cartoons and playing the games on their Nintendo Switch. Inside CTC Games, everyone is welcome to join in weekly social tournaments that run across three groups based on experience – from juniors and beginners to intermediate, masters and pro-league for adults. Brown says Pokémon is able to open up the lives of autistic children who are looking for connection. They want to belong somewhere, and with someone. As a game, Pokémon also plays to the strengths of many ND children whose focus and attention to detail means their ability to recall and remember facts and statistics is valued. The character designs and the conversations it sparks, as well as the competition it provides, all contribute to the success of CTC Games.

'What happens is they begin sharing an interest and socially interacting with each other.' He tells the story of a boy, aged six or seven, who came in with his mother a couple of years ago. 'He went straight to this box of ten-cent cards and focused on that. His mum brought him in because he loved Pokémon,' Brown says. But he would not interact, and Brown taught his mother how to play Pokémon. 'At the start, he wouldn't talk to me or acknowledge me or give me the time of day. Now he is asking questions and talking to me. His mum said just coming has greatly boosted his social confidence. He's almost a completely different person.'

Pokémon is the brainchild of Satoshi Tajiri who, as a teen, answered to the moniker of Dr Bug, growing up indulging his childhood passion of collecting bugs in a sleepy suburb in 1970s Tokyo. It was an area full of rice paddies, rivers and forests, a stone's throw from the growing metropolis. 'They fascinated me,' he told *Time* magazine in a rare 1999 interview. 'For one thing, they kind of moved funny. They were odd. Every time I found a new insect, it was mysterious to me, and the more I searched for insects, the more I found.' But soon the march of one of the world's big cities would swallow up his small suburb, which had clung to the edge of Tokyo, driving away Tajiri's insects. 'Every year they would cut down trees and the population of insects would decrease.' Later, as a teenager, arcade games became a fascination, and much later he developed Pokémon, which would go on to top the world's media franchises, overtaking Mickey Mouse and friends, Star Wars and Harry Potter.

For years, Tajiri has been celebrated as one of the world's big autistic brains; a claim allegedly spread early in a biography of the Pokémon creator and adopted widely across the media. Tajiri shuns media attention and has never commented. Suffice to say that Pokémon has been a game-changer for many: helping to prevent loneliness and develop connections; boosting teens' self-esteem, negotiating abilities and confidence in speaking; encouraging teamwork; and providing an outlet for competition.

CLUBS EQUALS CONNECTION

The importance of clubs, teams and pursuits based on interest cannot be underestimated for ND kids. In our research, the schools that hosted lunchtime or after-school activities – including many who had popular Pokémon and Dungeons & Dragons clubs – were able to provide stories of how children were able to build connections with their peers. As one mother told us: 'Dungeons & Dragons was the first thing my son showed a real interest in. Our goal was to steer him towards highly social hobbies, which would help him find like-minded friends. I enrolled him in online classes during Covid lockdown and he just loved it. Now that he knows how to play – he'll always be able to find a local Dungeons & Dragons group wherever he lives.'

Universally, we have been told by experts working with ND children that clubs and groups of like-minded teens are able to deliver connection that many might otherwise struggle to find. Not only can they help language development and encourage connections that feed friendships, clubs encourage teamwork and competition, and provide an avenue for a child to learn facial expressions, gestures and likely responses.

For a child who may find the classroom difficult, where a national curriculum takes centrestage, extra-curricular commitments can provide a valuable opportunity for connection. They can also encourage responsibility and help children to solve problems. Clubs boost self-confidence, providing opportunities for children to demonstrate leadership, get involved with public speaking and deliver a sense of achievement. Games such as Lego and Minecraft, for example, can also be used to develop social skills, and indeed therapies have been developed around some of those activities for autistic teenagers.

The list of activities doesn't stop at games. ND kids have limitless interests that can involve drama, musical theatre, scouts, girl guides, debating, languages, and any number of sports, hobbies or crafts, such as sewing or photography. It's not the choice of activity that is important but what it delivers, and for many ND teens this has proved revolutionary.

THE VALUE OF A TEAM

'[My son] did a program with St Kilda footy club called Saintsplay. The opportunity to play AFL with other kids who were ND or had other disabilities gave him so much confidence to play a sport and it was a safe environment,' his mother says. If a child 'was having a meltdown, staff didn't blink. If a kid put on their headphones, the staff would also put them on, so they were never alone,' she says. 'He is a typical autistic child; he doesn't do "team",' his mother says. 'But he learnt that he couldn't just take the ball and run. He had to pass the ball. He learnt to shake hands at the end of it. And because they were all similar, they didn't have to learn it off NTs – so there was no intimidation.' This year will be his fourth year with the club.

Alisa's twelve-year-old son has been playing tennis for seven years. 'He is an amazing tennis player and a better person for having such an amazing mentor. He turned his endless energy into good. We tried a few sports, but he wasn't necessarily great with team sports,' she says. Instead, her son has learnt routine and structure, and feels stronger after morning tennis training. And it started with an umpire seeing him swinging off a chair at the tennis centre. 'That guy who saw him swinging off the umpire's chair is still his coach. He got to know him and understand him and what motivates him and how to teach him.'

Many parents told us they had similar success when their kids joined Little Athletics, a program that is run in all states: 'Little Athletics has been great, and the volunteer coaches and other parents have been amazing. It's a good combination of structure and flexibility with an emphasis on personal growth and friendship. He may never win a race but he's made friends, listened to instructions and improved his gross and fine motor skills.'

Just as a single friend can make a world of difference, a teacher or coach can change a child's trajectory, helping them to translate their on-field skills to other areas of their life. Coaches, trainers and mentors can deliver lessons on the field, and those skills are then adapted off the field. As one parent told us: 'Our basketball coach now gives him one task to do each game, rather than expecting him to follow the play. It's worked really well, and he is now having small bouts of success, where in the past he wouldn't even touch the ball.' Another told us: 'My son has started basketball this year and has a lovely coach whose son is also on the team. My son went to a match a few weeks ago and was really anxious and started crying. The coach saw him upset and said that he can help her coach that day – fifteen minutes into the game my son asked her if he could play. It was the empathy and understanding she had for my son which I was so grateful for.'

Many parents said they experimented with a variety of sports before they found the right fit for their child. 'When my son was younger we started ninja gymnastics. The coach was amazing with him and explained to me that he himself has ADHD so understands how people can be judged unfairly or prematurely.' Another told us: 'A swimming lesson teacher who was a young male really took the time to find out about my son's interests, and then used them to engage him in lessons.'

> **'She has had a fantastic netball coach for the last few years, which has helped her develop some confidence outside the school arena.'**

The attitude of coaches and trainers is often critical for success, but as some parents told us, it is also an opportunity for ND children to engage with mentors who have autism or ADHD. As one mother noted: 'My daughter fell in love with dance early on, the structure and movement of ballet ticked all her boxes. One of her teachers asked her if she would do a ballet competition and believed in her. She wouldn't even walk in the classroom or on stage at assembly at the time, [but] she entered and came second. Now she is in a part-time professional program'. Another said: 'His taekwondo teacher is amazing with him. The teacher is also ADHD. [He] doesn't push him too hard, recognises when he is struggling emotionally, tells him it's okay and provides a story when a similar thing happened to him.'

Of course, not every child wants to join an extracurricular activity, and experts advise that if a child doesn't want to do an activity, they're unlikely to enjoy it or benefit from it. But the list of clubs is endless and there is ample choice for children to explore. Parents told us of success they'd had with cricket and drama clubs, and other clubs popped up too: chess and astronomy clubs, computer coding, skating and even playing in bands. With the affinity many autistic children have with animals, pony clubs have also become the passion for some; and research is ongoing into therapeutic horse-riding delivered to groups of ND children. Whatever the club, within short spaces of time parents could see their child 'fit in' and find a connection that had been difficult to make in the school yard. Success meant different things to different families, but in all cases the child benefited.

'Football coaches at our club have incredible belief in him and he thrives there. Many teachers put him down; the footy club builds him up. He is sixteen and now playing in the A-grade men's league.'

Boxing has also found a home in the lives of many young ND children who have energy to burn. Deuk Rae Kim, who goes by the name of Dundee Kim, is a two-time amateur boxing champion in South Korea and is perhaps best known in Australia for training former professional boxer Jeff Horn. Kim took up boxing to protect himself from bullies, later migrating to Australia where he became the founder of Dundee's Boxing and Fitness gym in Brisbane. He says boxing is able to strengthen a child's focus, direction and drive. Training was less about physical activity and more about 'motivation, persistence, education, encouragement, loyalty, growth and trust'. Kim says many autistic children struggle to 'cross punch' straight away, and teaching that also helped both their focus and their ability to communicate with their trainer. Younger children develop coordination and become more confident with eye contact as they 'toned up'. He sees himself in many of the young children who turn up, both ND and NT. 'I got bullied at school. I was a very shy boy and never looked into the eyes – especially of girls – in class!'

Cam Russell sees the same in the Modified Rugby Program (MRP) run by GingerCloud Foundation. Russell, who is the organisation's CEO, says the outcomes stretch far beyond the rugby field to embrace coaches and volunteers. The GingerCloud Foundation was set up by Megan and Anthony Elliott. They wanted to ensure their son, Max – who has a learning and perceptual disability – would thrive. 'For a while we had been asking ourselves how we could create a world where neurodiverse young people could live their best life,' Megan explains on the GingerCloud website. 'Where their individual successes would be celebrated, no matter how large or small. Where they could be part of, and contribute, to their community. Where the community would look for and experience what they can do, rather than focus on their disability and what they could not do.' And it has been a stellar success.

Russell says the program aims to embrace everyone, and currently has more female coaches than male coaches. Acknowledging that many ND young people have an issue with person-to-person contact, the biggest 'modification' is that players tag around the waist only. More than 300 children and coaches are involved in the program, which has five divisions, as well as 'player mentors'. These are drawn from two areas: firstly, mentors come from schools and clubs and join the GingerCloud community to help participants; and secondly, mentors are drawn from players who have moved through the ranks and who want to give back to the community that gifted them so many opportunities.

A feature of the GingerCloud program is a division of play for older teens who have been with the MRP for years, are bigger in stature, and who boast better-honed skills. That focus on growing up and embracing the future is strong. 'I want to transition them through to employment,' Russell says. 'Our program is more than a game.' The skills players learn are lifelong, including resilience and an ability to understand directions. 'We've got several young people who have done our program and then moved through to working in kitchens and customer engagement environments.'

Russell, who has coached and played rugby all his life, says he's never been happier in a work environment. 'To see the happiness of the parents and our young players ... you can't put a dollar value on it. It's more than the children playing the sport, it's seeing the really diverse demographics of parents uniting in one force on a Saturday morning or Friday night, on the sidelines.'

A FEELING OF BELONGING

Educator Sue Larkey says many school playgrounds offer no structure, and the rules that govern play can change constantly. For many ND children, a structure is needed to 'fit in' and create a sense of belonging. For example, she says, 'If you go to girl guides, there's a routine. You know who's going to be there. It offers a common interest, and it's normally supervised,' she says. Organised club activities also provide a connection, which underpins a sense of belonging children need. Larkey has this advice for parents: 'Don't do any spelling tests. Don't practise your maths. With ChatGPT they won't need any of that. But social connection is invaluable for resilience and belonging.'

> *'Scouts was a brilliant way to have a group of friends who didn't change and challenge him. He ended up earning the Australian Scout Medallion and going to the World Jamboree.'*

Larkey believes that social connection also helps to deliver emotional regulation. The value of a club that is separate from school allows children who can't find a connection inside the school grounds to know they are able to make friends elsewhere. Her call for action, though, extends back to schools. 'Schools need to set up clubs that come from a child's interests,' she says. Sending them out to the playground could be counterproductive. 'If you've got a child who loves Pokémon, set up a Pokémon club. If you've got a child who loves basketball, set up a basketball team.' Children will then have the opportunity to be part of a like-minded group.

And just in case some parents complain that those extra resources should go towards extension classes like maths, this is Larkey's response: 'Fair isn't everybody getting the same thing. Fair is everybody getting what they need in order to be successful.'

TIPS FOR JOINING IN

- Clubs and activities where teens meet others with similar interests can be a game-changer.
- Clubs can deliver a host of benefits including increased self-esteem, an ability to understand strategy and teamwork and read others' facial expressions, boost resilience, develop connections and develop new skills, like communication.
- Membership of a club, outside of school, provides an avenue for children to find others like them, outside of the classroom. This is good practice for all teens!
- Don't force your child to join a club but provide them with the opportunities so they know what is possible.
The range of clubs is enormous.
- Whether it's in person or online, clubs allow our kids to celebrate their interests, skills or knowledge, whether that's a Harry Potter club, Dungeons & Dragons, drama, music, basketball or chess.
- Schools need to be more proactive in offering lunchtime clubs. If your school doesn't offer any clubs, advocate for them. Many schools allow the kids to nominate lunchtime clubs each year from chess and crochet to art and book clubs.
- Go slow. Your ND child might like to sit and watch a club a few times from the sidelines before they're keen to participate.
- Having a friendship group outside of school means that when/if our school friendships go pear-shaped, we have other friends reminding us that we are likeable, seen and valued.

10. A FAMILY AFFAIR

EMILY PERL KINGSLEY SPENT FORTY-FIVE years – until her retirement in 2015 – writing scripts and songs for the beloved children's TV show *Sesame Street*. She received more than twenty Emmy Awards for her work on that iconic educational program alone. But it was her 1987 essay, 'Welcome to Holland', that cemented her popularity across the globe. Kingsley's son, Jason, has Down Syndrome, and in her essay, Kingsley explains that she is often asked to describe the experience of raising a child with a disability. She uses the analogy of a holiday – planning for a child is like planning for a dream trip to Italy. We might first buy a guidebook to develop our plan, then book a flight and pack our bags full of hopes and expectations, but when the plane lands, the hostess makes a shock announcement – we've arrived in Holland, not Italy. That's not what we signed up for, we think. But the flight plan changed, and Holland is our new holiday destination. Her point is this: Holland is not a horrible place, full of disease, famine and filth – it's just different to Italy. And while it is not what we were expecting, it is full of wonderful things, like windmills and tulips and Rembrandts. Even so, we hear people bragging about their Italy trip – the one we had planned. Kingsley finishes her essay explaining that the pain might not leave us, because our Italian dream holiday has disappeared. But if we fixate on that, we risk missing out on all the delights of Holland. (We've included, with her permission, Kingsley's essay on page 272.)

Speech pathologist Dr Bronwyn Sutton who works with ND children says, 'It's a lovely analogy for the journey [ND families] take.' She says that 'every individual is on their own journey of understanding'. Parents and siblings, aunts and grandparents will all take their journey of understanding at a different pace and in their own time. And when they work together, the family wraps its arms around a child with a disability, and things work out. But if they don't, it can be chaotic. It can cause terrible friction between parents, rivalries between siblings and misunderstandings within the wider family. When shame and blame dominate, everyone is swallowed up and starts squabbling over a child who needs all of their support and understanding.

As many parents told us, the journey of parenting a ND child has a number of challenges: as one mother admits, 'The key issue is not his autism – it's his lack of the essential skills needed in daily life. We can teach these with explicit repeated effort in a calm, positive, non-traumatising way, but this requires perfect parenting at all times – the pressure on the family is immense.'

> *'I'm a fighter. But I'm exhausted. We don't have any break of any description, ever.'*

Between them, Professor Tony Attwood and Dr Michelle Garnett have spent eighty years working with families who have autistic children. One of the most common questions they are asked is: 'Why is it so difficult to raise an autistic child?' Their clinical work shows that parents and caregivers of a neurodivergent child can face many obstacles that impact their physical health, psychological wellbeing, social network and finances. That is not in dispute. As we heard repeatedly during our research, many parents are struggling to cope. As one parent told us: 'I'm tired. I feel like society and the system is just grinding us down, when we are the ones needing more support.'

Other clinicians also raised concern over the load carried by parents, saying it could increase anxiety and cause nights of sleeplessness. Clinical psychologist Mary Kaspar says it has been shown that having a child with a disability is incredibly stressful, and means a couple is more likely to divorce. The challenges are also borne out in academic research. One 2023 study published in the *Journal of Autism and Developmental Disorders* involving sixty-six caregivers of neurodiverse children, showed challenges prompted by both the increased needs of the child and the lack of readily available support. Five problem areas were highlighted, including: barriers to community engagement; the impact on close relationships; the negative impact on mental health and identity; financial hardship; and a lack of identified support needs.

CREATING POSITIVE PARTNERSHIPS

Attwood says for parents, a diagnosis of autism or another neurodivergence can cause stress and the possibility of two different styles of child-raising might follow. He oversimplifies it for our benefit, but in many families the father might become the more authoritarian figure, with discipline at the ready. His partner might be full of love and acceptance of their newly diagnosed child. The parenting practices a couple may have adopted for other children may not necessarily work, and that can lead to friction – and inconsistency – about how to raise and discipline their ND child. Long delays in finding professional help might antagonise the situation, putting further strain on a marriage. Another catalyst that can confuse and sadden many parents is when an autistic child might not want to be hugged or not respond to expressions of love. Others struggle when extended family members might not believe the diagnosis, and judge parents for not implementing more household discipline.

'Parents can feel blamed and misunderstood rather than supported by extended family, and family rifts and resentment are common,' Attwood says. He says from his clinical experience, if the relationship is really strong, it will become watertight as couples share the load. 'But if the relationship is fragmented, it might tear it apart,' he says.

Attwood and Garnett suggest parents 'prioritise' their worries and problem-solve them with a support person. They have a long list of tips, which also includes staying connected, accessing good information, and looking after themselves in terms of nutrition, rest, exercise and spending quality time with each other. They also suggest writing an 'incredibly supportive letter' to yourself. 'Include in the letter the information you need to know on a daily basis, based on your knowledge of yourself, your child and autism, including any mantras that may help and any sources of inspiration, including heroes that you have, images, or quotes.' They encourage parents to 'make an appointment with yourself at the beginning of every day to spend two minutes reading this letter'.

Every clinician we spoke to made reference to the higher number of separations for couples who have a neurodivergent child. 'The divorce rate is extraordinarily high,' says speech pathologist Bronwyn Sutton. There is a strong view that married life takes on a new dimension when caring for a child with a disability, and this can be exhausting for parents. 'But the other [reason], which is not always talked about, is that the diagnosis brings with it an understanding that one of the parents might also be on the spectrum. And what happens, is that there's guilt or there's denial.'

Kaspar says that parents need to work together, and that begins and ends with the child coming first. In her clinical practice, she suggests parents use the Online Planning Tool created by Positive Partnerships to better understand the strengths and support needs of diverse learners. Kasper says this free online tool is easy to use and helps couples consider impacts and strategies, and therefore also assists communication. If the child has a secure attachment to their parents and is at the forefront of the couple's decisions, routines and strategies, it can be 'a really good outcome for the child'.

THE THREE-POINT PLAN FOR PARENTS

Author and parenting expert Dr Justin Coulson says he uses a simple model that helps parents achieve 'alignment'. The three-point plan encourages a couple to work together to approach an issue that is not working in the household. Each week, parents sit down together and ask themselves three questions.

1. **WHAT IS GOING WELL?** Coulson says this first question is crucial because we need to celebrate successes. 'And when you're raising kids in these circumstances,

sometimes it can be hard to do,' he says. Is it that your mornings have an established routine? Or one parent finds that they were more patient that week, and it had helped elicit a good response in their child. Or finding a child hates sitting at the table, providing a selection of foods and allowing them to pick at it worked well. 'Then double down on those things that are working,' he says.

2. **WHAT IS NOT GOING SO WELL?** 'It's a really simple question to ask, but,' according to Coulson, 'it's laden with grenades and bombs if we don't tread gently.' So, that means there needs to be rules – no blame, just observation. This could mean one partner might say they'd lost their temper too much. Or they both believed morning routines were chaotic. Or that their child refused physical activity. Or that screens have become an issue.

3. **AGREE ON AN ACTION PLAN:** This is where the couple look at one of those things on the list of things that did not work and decide, as a couple, which one to address. 'Just pick one,' Coulson advises. And try and 'get alignment on that one thing. It might be that we are struggling with the kids being unkind to each other. So, every night at the dinner table, we're going to talk to the kids about what was one thing that somebody did that was nice for you today. And what was one thing that you did that was nice for someone else today. Or maybe there's a screen issue and so we're going to sit down with the kids and work out a solution that we can implement as an experiment for a week and see how things feel.'

Essentially, if the couple can't agree on a firm plan of action, then they can agree to an experiment. 'For three days, we'll do it your way and for three days we'll do it my way,' he says. They both have to agree to be 'all in' and at the end of the experiment they assess what worked best.

The three-point plan is a strategy that will work effectively for couples who live together. For those who don't, Coulson says, 'Unfortunately, there's often animosity and an unwillingness to work together. There's underlying resentment, there's white-anting and all sorts of things. So, when that happens, my recommendation is that you treat your ex-partner like you would a client at work.' That means no angry, expletive-laden text messages — 'Because you wouldn't do that to a client, for example.'

Instead, Coulson suggests creating an online chat where you only talk business. 'Treat each other like business partners or clients, and take the same approach — here's what's working, here's what's not. And here's a struggle that I'm having.'

Of course, in reality, for kids in separated families there can be different rules around bedtimes, screen times and outdoor activities. 'And you might have an ex-partner who does not care one iota how much screen time kids get and what time they go to bed, and there's no such thing as outdoors because it just doesn't fit their lifestyle,' he says. 'When you are at that level of impasse, you simply accept that things are going to be different from one home to the other and there is nothing you can do about it. Stop fighting it because all the fighting only increases the animosity. The child becomes a living pawn in a power struggle between two adults.'

THE WORRIES KEEPING PARENTS UP AT NIGHT

A dominant fear that many parents face, particularly mothers, is thinking about the future. As one mum told us: 'I fear for my son as an adult. I can't even put it into words – how will he live? Will he need to be looked after? Who will be there to love him?'

The power of privilege also shone through in many responses. 'Mothers bear the brunt of diagnosis and care,' one parent told us. 'This is not surprising but can really suck. The system of diagnosis and support is easier for educated parents and people who can afford private services before NDIS funding. It continues the cycle of haves having and have-nots suffering. I'm privileged enough to have a job that I could do part-time in order to attend [my child's] therapy. But even when [I worked] full-time I had personal leave to be able to attend appointments. Many parents don't have this security and flexibility and the kids miss out.'

Most parents we surveyed reported exhaustion, struggling with differences in parenting styles, losing friends and feeling socially isolated. As one parent explained: 'I can't explain to you the work behind the scenes to support a "normal" day. He needs a snowplough parent to make everything easier and run interference when required. It's constant. He's not able to be independent at the same rate as other children. More broadly – it's hard to balance the time and attention he needs with my responsibility to my NT daughter – let alone work (I work full-time) or caring about anything else. Recently I had a friendship group of fourteen years dissolve (my daughters' mother's group) after one of the women said she was "sick of hearing about my autistic son" and then proceeded to tell me how to live and parent. I didn't know what to do. I can't accept the open judgement that my son is worth less conversation than other kids. So, I withdrew. But I really miss them. And my son misses them. Probably worse for me than the break-up of my marriage.' Another parent said: 'Divorce has been the hardest struggle. [My son] requires a lot of emotional support, care and patience with reflecting and managing behaviours and emotions. He gets, and trusts this, with Mum. He doesn't get this with Dad, which creates dysregulation in behaviour both at Dad's and at school after being at Dad's.'

Parenting can be difficult at any time – but the responsibility of raising a child requiring support can have drastic consequences for mothers, particularly. Repeatedly, we were told of an exhaustion and tiredness that meant many women had cut themselves off from friends or were no longer invited places. As one parent recounted: 'Loss of relationships with my sibling – who thinks my kids are a nightmare and "the best contraceptive ever" – my life-long best friend, other school parents. The list is endless. And exhaustion, unable to work so constant financial stress, school advocacy, battling the NDIS to the Administrative Appeals Tribunal, as they think my daughter can live independently!' We heard many similar stories: 'If you don't have a ND child and/or one with disability, it's incredibly hard for you to understand what it's really like to live with that child day-in, day-out and how hard it is to help that child. It is incredibly isolating for us as parents, as well as for the child. None of us is living the life we had thought we'd be living as a family. The only families who are willing to spend time with us have kids with their own issues, but that doesn't mean that the kids actually get on.'

Attwood says parents and carers need more understanding and less judgement. They might want to attend that book club, but just can't make it. They might eat takeout once a week to give themselves a brief break or decline a girls' weekend away simply because they can't leave their child. The anxiety some describe about their child's future prompts experts to encourage parents to seek counselling, too. While they are pivotal to their child's success they also need (and deserve) to live a fulfilling life.

SIBLINGS: THE GLASS CHILDREN

Raising a neurodivergent child often doesn't happen in a vacuum and can have a flow-on effect to other children in the family. As well as putting a strain on parents, it can also colour the relationship between NT siblings, and between NT and ND siblings. This can be magnified when one parent also has a neurodivergence, whether it is diagnosed or not. 'We've got parents who are incredibly stressed and stretched across many areas of their life. They're trying to be everything to everybody and there are added complications, especially if one of them is neurodivergent and hasn't ever had any kind of support,' Kaspar says. The focus on a ND child shouldn't mean less focus on their siblings. She says parents have to be really careful not to emotionally neglect a sibling.

In our survey, parents were aware that siblings often felt like 'glass children' – invisible next to the struggles of their brother or sister. One parent said: 'Both of them notice but she requires more from me as a parent and often a lot more leniency. As an example, my son started doing chores when he was eight. He now has three chores to do each week while my daughter has none. We have tried to implement chores for her but the mental gymnastics it requires for us as parents is too much, so it's a battle we have sidelined for now. Yes, it's unfair to our son – who is all about justice and equity – but he understands that our daughter sometimes requires more grace than he does.'

Another parent said: 'My daughter's life is forever changed by watching her brother meltdown, self-harm and threaten harm to those around him. I want you to know that our school systems (which I am absolutely a part of) are failing our ND kids. I want you to know that I love my child but every single day is hard and being a single mother who works full time as a head of department at one of the highest performing high schools in Brisbane sometimes feels impossible, but we have to keep a roof over our heads. I can't find a school that suits him and I'm relying on ageing parents in ill-health who are desperately trying to support me, but also don't understand autism or PDA.'

Kaspar says she sees the psychological impact – including anxiety, depression and obsessive compulsive disorder – that can occur in siblings of a neurodivergent child. Despite a parent's strong love, they might feel as if they are missing out or feel insecure within the family unit. 'Secure attachment' to their parents is an 'invisible kind of force' and they might not even be aware of how they are feeling, other than taking away 'the message that I'm unloved, I'm not important'. Kaspar's seen children then develop depression or become hell-bent on overachieving, or develop a belief that something bad is always around the corner. 'Emotional neglect can have massive consequences,' she says.

Attwood says siblings' confusion and even anger stems from their lack of understanding around autism. They wonder why their brother or sister is treated differently and subject to different household rules. One mother said: 'She hates her younger sister. My youngest adores her older sister and her older sister treats her appallingly.' Often, a sibling might also feel as though they can't talk to their parent as they might have otherwise. They might think they have enough on their plate already, and that they don't want to make life more difficult for them.

Jealously can also play a part. For example, if the family went to the zoo, but had to leave early because their younger brother was having a tantrum, a sibling might take that as their brother 'controlling mum and dad' when they wanted to stay longer. '[My daughter] and her older sister fight a lot; they are really different, and both get so frustrated at each other. I am struggling to help them overcome their differences and start to like each other again. I am doing my best; but it's bad.'

Sutton says that after an initial diagnosis, she often sees siblings go through an 'it's not fair' stage. They might believe their ND brother or sister is getting away with behaviour that would get them in trouble. Parents who approach this by educating the family in an open and honest way have more success, with siblings being able to appreciate that while things might not be 'fair' they can shift into what is called the empathetic stage. Sutton says, 'They start to advocate for their sibling and that's a beautiful thing to watch.'

Sutton has watched this play out many times in her almost forty years of practice. 'I've seen how often their siblings then take the empathy into their own careers and end up becoming therapists, nurses, and teachers – because they respect diversity.'

Kaspar believes that empathy is a crucial attribute for leadership. 'That's what we're looking for in leaders – people who are able to deal with all kinds of different people.' She points to the national education system and the current push for high ATAR marks. 'They've got that wrong. Leaders know how to include and work to support everybody's strengths and to treat everybody with respect. There's a movement in the leadership world that is about looking for those characteristics.'

Kaspar gives the delightful example of Jasmine Goon, who in Year 11 won the national 2022 Young Archies Award. Hosted by the Art Gallery of New South Wales, Goon took out the prize for her portrait titled 'And Who Shaped You?'

As her subject, Goon chose her younger brother, Kevin, who is non-verbal. She wrote in her artist statement: 'His brain has developed differently to a NT person. Despite my brother not being fully verbally communicative, he constantly inspires me to strengthen my integrity and acceptance of those around me. He, without words, has taught me how to develop approaches to other people's lives positively. Observing and growing up with him has taught me to not pass judgement on anyone, both inside and out.'

Psychologist Wesley Turner says he talks to parents and families about the importance of open dialogue, where siblings really understand the ND journey. 'I'm a big, big believer in attunement or synchrony,' he says. In laymen's terms, that means working towards understanding ourselves and those around us.

THE ND CHILD

The autistic child might not understand why their NT sister or brother doesn't want to spend time with them, or why they believe their lot is unfair. 'Theory of mind' is a core feature of autism, where an autistic child might have trouble understanding someone else's perspective. This can be a particular problem at home for their siblings. Tony Attwood says, 'Whilst all children are egocentric to some extent, the autistic child can take this to new levels, not because they are selfish or inconsiderate, but because they are not innately wired to consider how their actions and words may affect other people.' If the child is tired or upset, which can be often, it can affect other members of the family. 'Resentment can build over time with tense family dynamics occurring where both parties feel misunderstood and unhappy.'

Sutton says masking can also play a role here, because the more pressure a child feels, the more likely they are to mask. 'Sometimes children will mask more with a parent who they feel more pressured by.' She doesn't mean deliberate pressure is imposed by the parent. 'They might look up to their dad, and they want to be like their dad,' she says. 'So, you'll see a difference in the presentation to different parents, where they might let their mask down, or have more meltdowns in front of one parent.'

It can be a long hard road governed by schedules, routines and appointments that revolve around one child. For all members of the family, it can be lonely and exhausting, and impact everything from what a family eats, to the school holiday destinations they visit.

Burnout is real, and on every piece of advice we received, it was important – in some way – to take care of each other; to hold each other dear, talk openly and often, and know that working together will make family life easier for everyone, not just the ND child who is so often front and centre.

ADVICE FOR EXHAUSTED PARENTS

The stress associated with raising a child with additional needs is extraordinary. Some evidence suggests that when our emotional and cognitive resources are taxed, our willpower and our ability to be tolerant can diminish.

Parenting expert Dr Justin Coulson says that raising a neurodivergent child is 'one of the ultimate taxes on those resources'. Here's his top three tips for struggling parents:

1. As much as possible, work as a team. We've got to find people — family, friends and colleagues — to support us in helping our children.
2. Stop treating sleep as a luxury. If you want to be a better parent, sleep is essential. That means that you don't need to watch that extra Netflix episode tonight. 'You have to be at your best or you're going to feel like your world is falling down.'
3. The most important thing you can do for your neurodivergent child when it comes to their schooling is to be on the same team as their teachers. 'See them as an ally, recruit them, work with them and do everything you can to engender their support and to come across as reasonable.'

11. LIFE AFTER SCHOOL

THAT FINAL SCHOOL BELL, FOR almost every teen, signals a new beginning. Hats will be forgotten and stuffed with the unpolished shoes at the back of a bedroom cupboard. And the school bag, if it survives in any form, might be gifted to another student who is yet to feel the world opening up in front of them.

Many teens begin to reinvent themselves when they leave high school, free of the shackles that determined what they wore, where they sat, how their hair was fashioned and where and when they could speak. The irony of how modern schools operate in 2024 is jolting. On one hand, we tell our teens to be independent and think for themselves, we encourage them to pull their head out of the wallpaper of adolescence. But, on the other hand, we expect them to taper their personality to fit in with school rules and a one-size-fits all approach. Leaving school for the final time allows these young adults to escape to a new world and a much larger pool of peers. This can be difficult for kids as they try to find their own identity in a bigger sea of people, with fewer guidelines and restrictions.

School-leavers might find themselves navigating friendships without being enveloped in groupthink. Unscripted decisions can be made about what to wear and even when to wake up. Interests and passions grow alongside these new adventures, and for many ND teens this freedom can be liberating. Suddenly, they have the chance to pursue different career options, with apprenticeships and jobs, or to go to university or a trade college.

'Since starting uni they have actually improved their social connections, as the diversity of people is enormous,' one mother told us. For neurodivergent teenagers, it often unlocks a door; a point made by many parents whose child is about to, or has already, graduated. 'I don't hold as many fears anymore because I can see how well she knows herself, what she needs, and what she loves. She will still inevitably find our NT world tricky at times, but she is embracing her future options and is confident.'

> *'I don't have any fears, as I have been able to teach them how to succeed in the world. They will be amazing people.'*

Many parents believe if their child can graduate school, they'll flourish at university or TAFE where they can focus on their individual interests, without the unkindness of peers. 'I no longer fear for my child. She is grown, happy, studying at TAFE, in a relationship and thriving.' This is not an isolated comment and mirrors the journey of many NT girls, who often feel herded into friendship 'groups' they find stifling. As one mother told us: 'I think she will end up ruling the natural free world. We just need to survive school. She's street smart, savvy, strong, determined and stands up for herself. I wish I could be like her when I grow up!'

But no two journeys are the same; and for every child that relishes the freedom of leaving school behind, there are others who find the absence of school scaffolding challenging. 'The world is not built around her differences and she is expected to fit in. If accommodations are made, she could contribute so much, and her self-worth would soar.'

When the structures of school and home disappear, many older teens feel lost, their lives as chaotic as their bedrooms, and their planned tertiary study not working in the way they had wished. The need for advocacy and support post-school is strong. As one parent noted: 'I feel like we try [to] shelter them from the stigma that comes from being neurodiverse, but we can't hold their hands forever so we hope they will be okay.'

LOOKING FOR WORK

The number one fear that was identified in our research – by both parents and ND teens – is the fear of not being able to find employment. In the words of one parent: 'Finding a job is a big [concern] at the moment. Not being able to work in some settings due to anxiety limits what jobs are available. Not having a large network also limits connections to help find work.' Another agreed: 'We would like him to have a job over the Christmas holidays and are stuck with where to go, as normal teenage jobs won't work for him due to the sensory issues.' And this: 'I do worry about their job security, and I am working very hard to ensure I can leave them a good inheritance, so they are looked after.'

> *'I just don't know if he will be able to hold down a job.'*

Fears around children coping through the interview process and in the workforce were rife: 'How they are going to function in the working world worries me,' one parent told us. 'Many companies are just not educated enough or accepting enough of neurodiversity! People are just labelled as a bit strange in the workplace.'

Leaving school is one thing, but finding a job is another, and with it comes the inevitable hurdles of managing finances, working in a team, coping with a less structured timetable or tackling further study at university or TAFE. Until this point, parents have felt in charge of advocacy. But what happens next – when their child leaves home or obtains their driver's licence? And what happens after that, when parents get old and are no longer around? As one parent told us: 'Now he is seventeen, [his challenge] is finding a job and meeting a partner in the future. What will happen to him when I am no longer here?'

Employment is more important than providing a means for economic survival. Many of us judge our self-worth on the job title we have. It is also important in terms of providing purpose and routine, structure and a network of acquaintances that over time can morph into friendships.

If employment matches an individual's skills and values it can also deliver enormous joy, boost self-esteem and improve confidence. As one parent identified, their biggest concern for their son was 'finding a job that will engage him and challenge him'.

Problematically, the unemployment rate of people with autism sits at around thirty-four per cent; almost eight times higher than for people without disabilities. That's according to research involving workplace neurodivergence expert Dr Miriam Moeller from The University of Queensland. Other surveys suggest it might be much higher; for example, in one longitudinal study in the US, only fourteen per cent of ND participants obtained paid employment. The difference in the figures can be attributed to two main reasons: workplace involvement differs between ND people and capturing the data has been inconsistent. Either way, employment levels do not keep pace with the broader population, and often autistic workers are not employed in jobs that match either their skills or passions. Indeed, in our survey, employment was the number one concern of those parents or caregivers with an autistic child, just edging out concerns about dating and relationships, managing money, and a string of other concerns including impulsive behaviours that might lead to misadventure, a criminal record or death.

Children's author Kate Foster says the employment narrative around neurodivergence is not helped by common portrayals of 'all autistic people as geniuses', or lists that herald the top ten autistic entrepreneurs. Her point goes to the heart of any discussion about employment. If a brilliant autistic person wants to work for NASA, she says, they should be encouraged. But that's not for everyone. 'Why can't we just be normal?' she asks. Autistic achievers in history, such as Charles Darwin, Thomas Jefferson, James Joyce and Albert Einstein, are simply autistic achievers in history; they don't provide a script for all autistic people.

Foster's advice for young adults is to focus on their passion, and their comfort zone in doing it. 'I think the reason a lot of neurodivergent people go into the arts, and particularly stand-up comedy, is because you get to rehearse,' she says. 'One of the things that is very confusing for us is how we come across without looking weird and strange, because that's what we've been told so much.'

Practising and rehearsals mean lines and jokes can be worked and reworked, delivery honed and timed and even posture and presentation checked. 'It's the same in writing – I get to edit and edit and edit.' A writing career allows Foster to say exactly what she wants to say, how she wants to say it. 'It makes sense. It's a way for us to achieve the reaction and the result that we desperately want.'

Foster tells the story of an eighteen-year-old she met who was fascinated with people and human behaviour. 'So many neurodivergent people become psychologists and psychiatrists because, from such a young age, we are analysing people and their behaviours without realising it – we're trying to fit in and do what looks right and be the same as everybody else,' she says. The young woman asked Foster whether she thought it would be attainable for her to become a psychologist. 'Of course,' Foster told her. Most days can be carried on the back of belief, for almost anyone.

THE STRENGTHS OF A NEURODIVERGENT WORKFORCE

Austistic people face an enormous irony in seeking and maintaining work. No bar exists on those trades and professions to which an autistic person might aspire, and indeed many people only find out they are ND as an adult, when they are already high up the career ladder, or when their child is diagnosed. But the qualities often associated with autism – loyalty and reliability, attention to detail and focus, problem solving and identifying patterns that can highlight errors, as well as a strong sense of social justice and a preference for routine – are the specific attributes most valued by employers. So how can such a big gulf remain between what ND people can offer and the reality of lower employment rates?

Dr Leia Greenslade, an autistic academic teaching at Griffith

University, is the parent of a twelve-year-old who is homeschooled. Greenslade says that the local homeschooling community, like many others around Australia, is full of ND kids escaping mainstream schooling. They hold fears around their son's employment future because of the gap they see between rhetoric and reality. 'For those of us that do have stable employment, it can look to the outside world that we are very successful and thriving in our employment. The reality may be quite different, with many of us struggling to advocate for our needs in unsupportive systems.' Greenslade, who also supervises several PhD students undertaking research in the area of neurodiversity, says a rise in understanding the needs of ND people in the workplace is evidenced by the growing number of employee assistance programs. This is an acknowledgement that ND employees have valuable contributions to make.

'That said, it remains to be seen how effective these changes are in actually supporting ND people to find and keep jobs,' Greenslade says. 'Given that so many ND students are homeschooled, alternative pathways to employment are going to be needed.' Greenslade says while there was 'positive rhetoric around employment for ND people', sometimes it is nothing more than 'shiny words about inclusion and diversity' – ND workers are still expected to fit into a system that is unable to adapt to their needs. 'A good example of this might be creating a "sensory friendly space" in an area of a workplace but then expecting ND employees to be indistinguishable from their NT peers outside of that sensory friendly space. There are so many examples like this, where employers are saying all the right things in their recruitment packages, but in reality not

> *'Our fear has been unfounded – she got a job at Macca's.'*

being interested in addressing systemic inequalities in practice.'

Pip Williams, author of the best-selling novels *The Dictionary of Lost Words* and *The Bookbinder of Jericho*, is also a social scientist with a PhD in public health. At fifteen, Williams discovered she was dyslexic. Her early teachers signalled a problem with her spelling, and she was told to improve her focus and concentration. Her written work rarely reflected what she knew. Later, a teacher sought alternative ways of assessing her ability. For example, her written work was accompanied by a sit-down discussion that carried weight. It unlocked a door that has allowed Williams to follow her passion, develop a strong career and find contentment.

So, what's her answer to encouraging a dyslexic child to write?

'That's easy,' Williams says. 'Never mark their spelling.' Spelling is just a tool in word use; the real power of words is in their meaning. 'I can give you so many examples of words that have been arbitrarily spelt in the dictionary because no one could decide on the best way to spell them,' Williams says.

After all, she says, if Shakespeare could misspell his own name, why do we put such stock on the individual letters in words? 'If a child hands you an assignment or a birthday card – focus on the ideas and creativity in that piece of work and don't for a second spend any time correcting,' she says. 'Just engage with the ideas and the creativity – later on, you might remember where they were having trouble with their spelling and that might become part of a lesson down the track, but don't associate the mistakes with the thing that they've done, which is creative – that's just negative reinforcement and you're essentially punishing them for doing something creative and thoughtful.'

As Williams climbed through school, she honed in on her

creativity and uncanny ability to tell a story. It made a lifelong difference to Williams, who says that writing 'was the only way' she could express herself. 'I've met a lot of people who stopped writing because they were criticised for how they did it – and I think that's a terrible shame.'

For the record, Williams still struggles with spelling. 'Dyslexia doesn't necessarily go away,' she says, but a dyslexic brain also delivers impressive strengths. Her success as an author is perhaps the best testament to this; *The Dictionary of Lost Words* is now a *New York Times* bestseller and was the first Australian novel to be selected for Reese Witherspoon's book club.

'Dyslexic brains are very good at making connections where ordinarily a connection can't be seen, which means you can be very creative and a good problem-solver. British intelligence agencies hire dyslexics because they are very good at code breaking.'

THE DIGITAL ECONOMY

Geoff Smith, the CEO of Australian Spatial Analytics, believes that many autistic people ply their skills in the digital economy and go on to become rockstar employees. A data analyst and former disability employment executive, Smith's TedxBrisbane Talk called 'Autistic minds are primed to become rockstars of our big data economy' is well worth a listen. Smith advocates for social enterprise to be the vehicle to unlock ND talent pools for big organisations and corporations, because he saw how the system of supporting people to get off Centrelink and into general employment wasn't working. He said this was particularly the case for autistic people. 'We would place them into jobs where they just weren't thriving.' That proved the impetus for the

2020 birth of Australian Spatial Analytics, which is now one of Australia's biggest social enterprises, boasting a workforce where seventy-five per cent of employees are autistic. With 300 employees, its hope is to grow to 1000 by 2030.

Smith says he has learnt a swag of lessons from his growing ND workforce. The ND mind often shines when tasked with technical issues, and his workplace was filled with employees with remarkable attention to detail, an interest in technology and a range of skills, including logic, memory, intense focus and pattern recognition. 'That's all super important for the skills shortage we have in Australia,' he says.

The notion that ND employees can excel if they are working in a supported environment is not surprising. Nor is the fact that Smith's employees love starting the day knowing what they would be tasked with. Smith identified early that this structure was crucial to workers' comfort levels. But while every worker is different, with a unique personality, together they create a culture that allows the team to perform at high levels.

Smith says, 'They think differently to NT minds, they have different ideas, different kinds of interests, both socially and culturally. And so that melting pot creates an awesome and vibrant place to work. The energy that a group of ND minds can contribute to anywhere in society, whether it's a workplace or not, is quite special and a bit hard to quantify.'

Smith admits that the comedic talent of many of his staff also helps. 'They're bloody funny – from the lighthearted humour to the self-deprecation. Very quick witted,' he says of his team. And he's learnt that many have awesome debating skills, are able to think on their feet and respond with lightning speed. Of course, there are challenges. 'It's not all sunshine and rainbows,' he says. Different communication styles and tolerances to social interactions can lead to misunderstandings around context and body language. A host of small adjustments have also helped to improve comfort levels for his staff – many of whom routinely wear headphones – and include turning down office lighting, muting strong sensory inputs and relocating noisy air-conditioners.

Q&A with Anthony, aged twenty-four, who has ADHD and autism

Q: When you left school, what did you hope to do?

A: *I wasn't sure what I wanted to do at that point, I always wanted to work in a creative field, but I dropped out of high school at fifteen due to mental health issues. Four years later I went to film school, but then started work at Australian Spatial Analytics after that.*

Q: Have you met friends at work?

A: *I have made several friends through work, both in Brisbane and Melbourne.*

Q: Describe the job you do at ASA?

A: *I'm a Lead Data Analyst and Project Manager for an ongoing project with one of our biggest clients. The work we do in my project is telecommunications engineering for NBN installations, using GIS software to design new networks and produce 'as-built' packages for NBN to update what has been done in-field, after the fact. My role in the project has included scoping the work, training on-site with the client, training new analysts on*

> the project, the day-to-day operations of managing workload, communicating with the client, with either technical queries or clarifying delivery processes and finances. As a Lead Data Analyst, I also manage the people in my team as a direct manager, providing support and mentoring as well as managing shifts.
>
> **Q:** What is important to you in your work environment?
>
> **A:** *I like to have friends in the office to interact with, as well as plenty of challenging work to engage me... Also working in an office is very helpful to me, as doing any sort of work at home I find extremely difficult.*
>
> **Q:** What would you say to other neurodiverse young adults who are looking for a job?
>
> **A:** *I never thought I could work in this kind of office environment, and certainly never expected to be in leadership/management. But, given the right environment, I think neurodiverse people can excel beyond neurotypical people in this kind of work, so you shouldn't feel like it might make working harder.*

LANDING A JOB

Smith says 'getting in the door' is the biggest challenge for most people entering the workforce, and for young ND applicants the interview process, especially, can be a challenge because they don't necessarily understand social cues or follow an expected social script. 'My advice for young people looking for a job is to try and find that alternative pathway by harnessing your strengths. See yourself as an asset. See your condition as an asset. And then don't be afraid of the life-coaching you may need prior to employment or during employment. That kind of scaffolding is important.'

Jasmine Parker is head of people and culture at AMAZE, an Australian autism organisation, which was originally set up by parents looking for more resources. Before a resumé is completed, Parker suggests ND jobseekers sit down and make a list of their strengths that could be transferable to a work context. She suggests this is done with someone they trust, so that they discuss it and seek objective feedback.

Jobseekers should then consider the workforce environment by searching job boards they trust. What kind of jobs are out there? What kind of skills and experience are employers seeking? This second stage allows the jobseeker to create a shortlist of their strengths and how they might match specific jobs on offer. Can the jobseeker imagine themselves in this role? Is the job at the one building, or does it change location regularly, which might be more challenging? What reasonable adjustments might they need to be successful in the job they are considering? It might be noise-cancelling headphones or adaptive technology, for instance. 'Try to create a list based on what you can offer, and what is going to work,' she says.

Once that is done, and there is an alignment between the jobseeker's strengths and interests and the role being offered, it's time to work on a CV. Similar to most CVs, ND jobseekers should include a personal profile, outline the strengths and characteristics they can offer in the role, and record key skills and knowledge, along with education and work experience or volunteer history.

The job interview also involves preparation. Parker suggests jobseekers contact the organisation before the interview. What reasonable adjustments can they offer ahead of the interview?

Can questions be sent in advance? Can the interview be conducted in a quiet space, or even online? Other questions might relate to who is conducting the interview, the names and titles of anyone else on the panel, the length of the interview and its format. For example, is it a competency-based interview or a task-based interview?

Answers to these questions, ahead of an interview, can reduce anxiety, Parker says, but it also allows the organisation to consider its inclusivity opportunities.

Ahead of the interview, Parker suggests jobseekers start role-playing interviews. Practise asking follow-up questions that are a feature at the conclusion of interviews and consider ways to demonstrate knowledge that will add value. For example, if the jobseeker was asked about a project, they could explain how it was successfully completed, but also their reflection on any improvements that could be implemented. If questions aren't provided in advance, the job description will always help narrow down likely avenues for discussion.

'I see a shift to a more inclusive world for ND people and I'm confident they will find their place in the world.' That's the response of one parent, whose child is now lining up for a job, along with their NT peers.

Smith believes we should all share in that hope too, partly because of the growing recognition of autism, the increasing role of autistic workers in advocating for themselves, and a new willingness of people, as adults, to seek out their own diagnosis. Smith's hope runs beyond that. He says even discussions of neurodiversity on the front page of newspapers, while not always carrying the tone they should, are an opportunity to educate others, including employers, about the opportunities for workers – but also workplaces.

AIMING HIGH

Many with lived experience of neurodivergence are hopeful that inclusivity in the workforce is changing for the better. Take, for example, April Lea, a high-performing engineer in the tech industry who was diagnosed with ADHD and autism at the age of twenty-seven. In 2021 she was included in Hot Topics' Top 100 Emerging Engineering Leaders. That same year, she suffered severe burnout and spent a month in hospital, followed by a six-month hiatus from the workforce. This prompted a decision to relook at her lifestyle and consider if she wanted to sustain the same levels of performance. April knows what it is like to encounter discrimination and stigma: 'I'm a very capable technology leader; I've been in the industry for more than ten years,' she says. 'In an interview at a medium-sized technology business I was asked, "How can you be an effective leader with autism?" I said my results speak for themselves.' This experience prompted her to launch The Safe Space Collective – an online platform that provides education, advice, tools and strategies for HR teams and leaders to embrace and manage neurodiversity. 'Workplaces are getting better,' Lea says. 'The empathy and awareness is definitely improving.'

Ample evidence reveals that ND employees add to the bottom line. At SAP, a multinational software corporation, workers including autistic employees have been credited with technical fixes that saved US$40 million. Multinational finance company JPMorganChase found their ND employees to be forty-eight per cent faster and ninety-two per cent more productive than their NT employees. That sort of success, across companies and industries, doesn't surprise Bodo Mann, the CEO of auticon Australia and New Zealand, which forms part of the biggest autistic IT consulting businesses in the world.

Employing more than 465 autistic people in fifteen countries, auticon was formed in 2011 by a German entrepreneur whose son was on the spectrum. Mann says it was set up as 'a little bit of an experiment; he set it up as a social enterprise'. Less than fifteen years later, it operates across the globe. Mann is direct about the challenges ahead. He says he wishes Australia would embrace neurodiversity more, in terms of how it is perceived in the community and the support provided by government. He notes that many other countries, including the UK, Germany, Norway, Denmark and Sweden, are ahead of the Australian corporate sector, which doesn't always appreciate what neurodiversity could bring to the table.

Employment of ND workers is not about 'doing the right thing' or 'having social impact', he says. While this is important, for-profit ventures can also create real value through new innovation and productivity. Mann says that innovation is widely seen as a product of different cognitive strengths and different ways of viewing problems; in short, a team of different people. 'By definition, autistic talent does that,' Mann says. 'They are very different in the way they attack a problem from a NT individual.' Their wide skillset – ability for hyper focus, strong concentration over long periods, and recognition of patterns and errors – is invaluable. So is a brutally honest and direct communication style, which is regarded as a benefit in the corporate world, where meetings are to the point, focused and run on time. In addition, few ND employees wasted time on corporate politics.

In 2024, auticon helped autistic racing car driver Ben Taylor by providing analytic support looking at his on-track data. Its autistic data analysts and software engineers were deployed to build insights that were aimed at taking Taylor's driving to the next level. Taylor was diagnosed as autistic with ADHD at seventeen and believes it has delivered him unique strengths that help his track performance. His message for other young adults: find your strengths and believe in yourself.

Mann says he recruits autistic talent who are usually a few years older than school leavers. 'They don't have to have a degree, but we look for a passion for technology, and also the ability to work as part of a team environment.' As outlined elsewhere, some autistic workers can struggle in team environments, but others embrace it. 'So, they don't have to play football, but a lot of them actually do like to interact as part of the gaming environment,' Mann says. Building those skills, like interactive muscle, allowed workers to converse with both clients and fellow team members.

Mann's advice to jobseekers is the same as other experts in this area; focus on a passion, which might be technology or driving or baking. Some experts suggest teens undergo a detailed assessment during high school to try and focus on talents and passions to better identify a career path. And then grow your talent. Fertilise it. Nurture it.

'Ben Taylor didn't wake up and say, "I'm going to be the best racing driver in the world," Mann says. He needed to build a tangible capability by investing time and effort. That might include focusing on those skills that can be challenging, such as teamwork, or overcoming setbacks when applications are not successful or jobs prove to be the wrong fit.

Coaches are used widely at auticon to both address workers' mental health and ensure technical proficiency. Social skills can also be targeted. While the use of coaches helps in developing a friendship toolkit and building resumés, social skills and timetabling, this should not be seen as exceptional. Many people have mentors, whose role is to challenge us, help us identify our own talents – and weaknesses – and encourage self-growth.

A mentor or coach who also has a neurodivergence could also be a spectacular asset to any teen's team. ADHD coach Tamara Rosier says she can see a generational shift in how young workers were approaching the employment market. 'The youngest ones will just declare, "I have anxiety, and I have depression and maybe an eating disorder." It's kind of in your face [when they ask]: What are you going to do about it?' Slightly older workers, in their thirties and forties, also believed the workplace should accommodate for them. But she cautions against unadulterated optimism. In her experience, she says, workers with ADHD and other conditions can be punished for trivial issues, like turning up seven minutes late. She advocates for both personal and environmental responsibilities. 'We have to do both. We want the work environment to help. We also want you to learn not to mask your symptoms, but to accommodate for yourself too.'

Q&A with Harrison, aged twenty-three, who has Asperger's and ADHD

Q: What is important to you in your work environment?

A: *As long as there is something new to learn, I'll be satisfied. Otherwise, the days will seem long and I'll get restless with more of the same. And less bright lights are always preferred, but not necessary.*

Q: Have you found discrimination in the workplace in other jobs?

A: *When I applied for my first couple of jobs and listed autism as a disability, I was asked if it would impact my ability to do the job. This was always very demoralising. Eventually, I stopped doing this and noticed that I was treated much differently than before.*

Q: Were you nervous about any interview, or how did you prepare?

A: *I was nervous about my interview. It was the first time that I was ever interviewed for a role that I actually wanted, rather than to just pay the bills. To my surprise, they provided the interview questions in advance, and I was able to prepare with a lot less anxiety.*

Q: What would you say to other neurodivergent young adults who are looking for a job?

A: *As tempting as it is to mask your behaviours to increase your marketability in the job market, it's very exhausting and isn't a viable long-term strategy. If you have the opportunity, keep looking for somewhere that accommodates you and your needs rather than you trying to accommodate for them.*

Q: If you had a tip for someone in Year 11 or Year 12 who is worried about finding a job, what advice would you give them?

A: *Your advantage is your age. Put your hand up for as many opportunities and experiences as possible. It helps build your resumé and build your understanding of what you do and don't enjoy doing. With each day that passes, the chances of getting a job increase.*

POST-SCHOOL STUDY

This chapter has really focused on finding work, because that elephant gets bigger in the minds of ND students and their families as the end of high school looms. But that in-between period for many students, where they take on a trade or pursue vocational or tertiary studies, can also be a difficult time. Certainly, school doesn't prepare students for some of the challenges they face in the job arena or the university classroom. As one parent noted: 'There needs to be advocacy for supports at university level, too. I work in a university and the tertiary institutions have diabolical processes to navigate. I imagine it would come as a shock to a child who came through a supportive primary and secondary experience.'

That comment will not surprise parents who have a child leaving school. Whether it's extreme scaffolding, which has grown at big private schools determined to graduate the brightest, or a lack of planning on behalf of students and parents, employment has now become a significant issue, post school. Some educators put it down to Covid, or to parental mollycoddling. Others attribute it to the surge in anxiety we have seen in adolescents. But what it means is that a chunk of school-leavers graduate high school without the skills to grow their independence as they celebrate becoming an adult. They may lack financial literacy, an ability to cook, skills for washing and ironing their own laundry, and struggle to get their driver's licence. University lecturers see it daily on campus. Teens missing classes because they forgot or were not used to using an alarm. Others with no understanding of an assignment process that didn't include several 'feedback' opportunities granted by teachers.

Different timetables each day can present challenges, along

with different student cohorts. Even deciding what to wear, after years of uniforms, can pose a challenge. These issues can be significantly harder for a student with a neurodivergence. This surfaced repeatedly in our research - the 'huge black hole' a young person could fall into after the structures of school collapsed. As one parent told us: 'When the structures of school and possibly home were removed, my daughter really struggled with many aspects of uni life: living away from home; using different academic systems; keeping on top of content and assignments without the close interaction of teachers; having to manage time and prioritise. Some uni lectures were very long – [it was] hard to focus for that length of time and hard to process a huge dump of information. At uni, no one calls you into account about missing lectures or tells you to pre-read stuff, or revise content and prepare you for exams. She failed miserably in a number of units. She was also trying to balance study with a couple of part-time jobs. Living on campus in a college was a challenge too – a lot of distractions, noise, activity, less than ideal food (no one to make sure she ate meals). She ended up leaving uni and taking a gap year.'

Some parents noted that their children were dealing with work, but other life skills were lacking. One parent said their daughter had a part-time job and was managing well, 'However, the adulting part of life is less smooth, things like keeping track of appointments, medications and when they are going to run out, eating and cooking for herself, accessing therapy outside of crises. She still needs a fair amount of support from us, both financially and emotionally, with day-to-day adulting tasks.'

In another case, an eighteen-year-old asked his mother whether he could seek a diagnosis in October of his first year at university. She visited him, an hour up the road from where she lived. His room was a mess. His books sprayed across the room. He hadn't been to lectures for three weeks. 'Mum, I need to come home. I don't know what's happening,' he told her. Following an ADHD diagnosis, he is now back at university. 'And I cannot believe it – he's a changed person,' his mother says. 'Focused. Interested in his study.' The last time she popped in, his room was significantly tidier.

Clinical psychologist Tony Attwood says autistic students need to advocate for their own style in tutorials. The week before our interview, he had a university client he has known almost her whole life. 'She was having difficulty in tutorials,' he says. She wanted to contribute, but the pace moved too fast. She would be asked a question, and by the time she was ready to reply, the class had moved on. He suggested she choose the right time to tell them she was autistic and this meant she might need to think more about her response before providing it. 'So please, if you ask me a question, just wait, and I will answer you.'

Planning for university or further study – especially for ND students – needs to start early. As post-school planning isn't delivered at high school, it needs to be taken up at home. What does your child want to do when they leave the school gates for the last time? And how can you embed the skills needed be taught, step by step, as they traverse their teen years? Often, and perhaps because of those support structures at home and at school, the same lessons apply for all teens. Do they understand financial literacy? Consent? Are they able to cook ten basic meals? Do they know how to develop their own routine, even if it means carrying a laminated note in their pocket to remind them? Are they committed to their own welfare, in terms of diet, exercise and sleep? The list is long, and specific challenges will be harder for ND students.

TIPS FOR ND JOBSEEKERS

Jasmine Parker, head of People and Culture at AMAZE, provides the following advice for ND young people when they are considering entering the workforce for the first time.

- Sit down and list your strengths that could be transferable to a work environment. Do this with someone else – either someone in your family or a trusted friend – so you can have a discussion from an objective viewpoint and take on feedback.
- Search trusted job boards to find out what the market looks like: What jobs are on offer? What skills or experience are in demand? This allows you to match your strengths with specific job descriptions. This should also include consideration of any reasonable adjustments that you might need in the workplace.
- When it's time to write a CV, align your strengths with the job being advertised. Like any CV, it should include a personal profile, strengths and characteristics, key skills, knowledge, experience, education and work volunteer history.
- Before any interview, seek information: Are the questions available ahead of time? Where will the interview be held? By whom? What type of interview is it?
- With that information at hand, it's important to role-play scenarios so you can confidently answer questions and also ask follow-up questions of your potential employer.

12. DATING AND DRIVING

IN A PUB IN NEWCASTLE, 160 kilometres north of Sydney, a long table has been set up. It could be any night of the week at any Australian pub, as a crew of young people enter through the front door in dribs and drabs. But tonight is the inaugural Match Mate initiative – an opportunity for ND people to speed date, or simply to make connections and develop friendships after leaving school – in recognition that this can be an isolating time for young adults.

Georgia Ostler, a twenty-five-year-old occupational therapist, is helping the two organisers by laying cards on the table to prompt conversation between the twenty-three ND young adults who have turned up; many with their support workers. Because communication can be difficult, the cards are filled with social stories to help break down how the evening will work. For example, pictures of the organisers are strewn along the centre of the large table letting people know whom they can ask if they have any questions. Everyone has a name tag on and has been asked to come prepared to introduce and nominate a fun fact about themselves, as a way of breaking the ice. When Georgia kicks the evening off, she introduces herself and tells the group she plays rugby. As the rest of the table take turns, it becomes clear that they share strong mutual interests, with many participants enjoying cars and video games.

Making use of the conversational prompts, the group asks simple, inclusive questions to get the ball rolling. What is your favourite part of the day and why? Would you rather live by the ocean or live by the mountains, and why? If you won the lottery, how would you spend it? If you could be granted three wishes, what would they be?

> *'I want her to find her autism profile and understand who she is, and for her to love herself. She's such a bright light and I don't ever want her to lose that.'*

Organisers watch as connections are made and grow. At first, eye contact is limited and conversation restricted to short, direct responses. But before long, elements of humour and sarcasm are introduced as the group start to feed off each other. 'It was actually incredible,' Ostler says of the changed atmosphere. 'Unprompted chats, genuine laughs – connection and communication that you don't typically see otherwise.' By the end of the night, 'people were giving out their numbers to catch up with each other!'

Dating and driving, like finding a job, are rites of passage for older teens as they develop the independence that delivers them into adulthood with the skills to manage their own lives. But navigating early adulthood can be downright hard. When it comes to dating, many ND young adults might face a range of challenges including an inability to read social cues and body language. They might struggle to understand the nuance of what someone might be saying. Just like the rest of us, they want to fit in, are vulnerable and loyal, but will have to face conflict, sex and issues around consent.

Those big, exaggerated feelings that trip up most people during their first romances were also cause for concern for many of the parents we interviewed. As one parent told us: 'I'm not looking forward to dating and heartbreak. My child is seventeen and I have managed to steer them away from emotional experiences. This will be deep felt and potentially very dramatic.' And: 'She's so big hearted and empathic. I worry her heart will be broken and she's going to feel it so very deeply. It's happened a number of times with friendships but romantically will be a huge tragedy.' Another parent agreed: 'He is going to be very tall and I worry once the hormones kick in he will lash out and hurt someone or be hurt back. He's such a lovely kid, but once he has a meltdown he can't control [himself].'

SEX, PORN AND CONSENT

Cath Hakanson, a sex educator from Sex Ed Rescue with over twenty-five years' experience, says it's crucial for parents to 'keep the door open, so kids know they can come and talk about all the stuff they're hearing about'. Social media could be an ally here, providing opportunities to prompt discussions. 'The more we can talk about this stuff, the more it sort of buffers and protects our kids.' That's her first point. The second is to use resources that are available, including the plethora of books and online assistance around sex education. 'It's about being factual and then talking about consent, talking about the fact that sexual feelings can be really big feelings, and they can be really overwhelming as well.'

No topics should be off the table, including masturbation. 'I'm getting a lot of parents coming to me whose kids are starting to develop fetishes from a young age with masturbation.' Hakanson provides the example of autistic children who have found park swings and other equipment arousing. What's the impact of another, perhaps younger, child seeing that, and police being called? It's her question, and points to a simple lesson that needs to be articulated: that sex acts are private and should be done in the privacy of a home. Hakanson says numerous cases exist where ND children start acting out sexually in public, even ending up in the court system. Later, she says, it is discovered that they'd not received any early sex education. It's a plea for diagnosis. 'Diagnosis is a privilege. You've got to have money to be diagnosed, and you've got to have a parent who cares enough to pursue it.'

We've made the point repeatedly that no two ND teens are the same, as no two NT teens are the same. In terms of dating: trust the knowledge you have of your own child. Usually, parents know their children better than anyone else and that expertise needs to be used to navigate tricky areas. What are the traits our children have that they might need to focus on improving in coming years, and what resources might help? Encourage conversations, watch television shows and access online resources, podcasts and books around the topics. For example, if they are impulsive in decision-making, it's important to talk about the steps that lead to consent. 'Make sure you have a conversation that fits in around those traits,' Hakanson says.

Hakanson is aware that women are vulnerable to sexual assault. Girls often feel pressure from their peers to fit in and others are susceptible to grooming. 'Young ND teens in a relationship might not think through their sexual decisions and might do stuff that they will then regret.' This was confirmed by parents, when asked what they were most worried about. 'Teen dating. Having poor emotional regulation is difficult in relationships,' said one parent. 'Sex abuse,' said another. 'People with disabilities face disproportionately higher rates of abuse.' These were not isolated answers, with one parent saying they were worried about their child 'being assaulted and not being able to tell me'. Another worried that, 'she will end up in an abusive relationship'.

Sadly, evidence underscores their concern. Experts are familiar with this issue in their own practices, with broken-hearted daughters, often with supportive parents, trying to navigate a way forward after an assault. In a 2016 study conducted by Sarah Bargiela, Robyn Steward and William Mandy on the 'Experience of Late-Diagnosed Women with Autism Spectrum Conditions' nine out of the fourteen participants reported sexual abuse. Half of these happened inside a relationship where women felt obliged or were 'pestered' into sexual activities. The study showed how young autistic women were vulnerable to sex abuse. 'I kept trying to break up with him, and whenever I did, he would say I didn't know my own feelings … I felt so trapped.'

Clinical psychologist Wesley Turner again reiterates how important it is for teens to tap into how they are feeling on the inside. His conversation with a young person might go like this:

ADULT: What did you feel like in that situation?

TEEN: He came and hugged me.

ADULT: Did you want to be hugged?

TEEN: No.

ADULT: For how long did he stay hugging you?

TEEN: A long time and he pressed up against me.

ADULT: Don't worry about if you could or not, but what did you want to do at that point in time.

TEEN: I wanted to punch him in the dick.

Turner will then explore why she didn't listen to that internal message in the moment. 'And then we'll dive into the context. What could you do if something like that happened again so that you listen to your own anger? What would you do if he asked for a hug in the first place? It's about determining how to not get into a situation, which is almost impossible, in some cases. But then how to respond to it – how to react during, and after, the fact.' It's advice for all our teens, not just young adult women.

Indeed, parents also expressed fears about their sons experiencing big emotions, falling in love, not reading cues, following what they've seen online, and not what is in their heart. 'Dating will be tough,' one parent said. 'He is an overthinker who will read more into situations than there is.' Others worried that their boys may not really understand consent or may not be able to read the nuances of body language, contexts and comments.

The concern of parents, whose children begin a relationship, is not confined to the ND community. How many of us have stayed awake, but pretended to be asleep when our children arrive home from their first date? But the risks for those with a neurodivergence is greater. Hakanson provides context here, saying impulse control might be improved by medication, 'but kids don't always take medication. They might take a break during the school holidays or on weekends,' she says. Again, it comes back to ongoing, regular and persistent conversations. 'You can't change your behaviour if you're not aware of what is happening,' she says.

If teens are aware of their impulsivity, it lays the groundwork for teaching self-awareness or to question their decisions as they make them. Hakanson isn't suggesting this is easy; just necessary. Parents can help by leaning into these conversations. Windows of opportunity to talk about these issues will surface constantly, particularly at the start of a romantic interest, and before it becomes sexual. 'You need to talk about how a relationship develops,' she says.

Hakanson recommends books written by autistic romance authors that detail how you might know if someone likes you or not. 'They share their uncertainties. They share the struggles with communicating and misinterpreting body language. And that stuff is so valuable, because most other romance books don't talk about it – you just "know" that someone likes you.' She says TV dramas, while good for prompting discussions about dating and relationships, don't always show the indecisiveness and reluctance that often occur in intimate relationships, and just watching shows can make it harder for many young adults to notice these behaviours and learn from them.

> '**My child has one year of school left and we have no idea what happens next.**'

Autism experts Michelle Garnett and Tony Attwood describe some of the many strengths an autistic partner can bring to a relationship. 'An autistic partner may have a mind that can grasp astonishing complexity, they may be wonderfully attentive, have deep compassion, be fair-minded, very talented in their field, extremely loyal or different in ways that are intriguing but not yet fully apparent.' However, if their partner is neurotypical, issues that are perplexing can arise. 'We have learnt through our vast clinical experience that approaching relationships between autistic and non-autistic individuals can be likened to a cultural exchange program, where there needs to be understanding and acceptance of each person's "culture" for the relationship to succeed.' That is true in all relationships but plays out more significantly when one partner in the relationship is neurodiverse, and specifically, autistic.

'Theory of Mind' explains an ability to read someone else – their expressions and body language. As we know, because autistic people can find this difficult, it can be hard for the NT party to read the thoughts of their partner. This is the 'double empathy problem' in play. As Attwood and Garnett explain, 'the autistic partner may seek solace in their passionate interest or in solitude to recharge their energy levels. While an autistic partner may totally understand this need, a non-autistic one may feel neglected and wonder why their partner is not choosing to spend time with them.'

Like all partnerships, other issues pop up based on differences: the exhaustion of social engagements, differences in the amount of time they want to spend together, different communication styles and even the delivery of comments. Was that funny? Or sarcastic? An autistic person may be so focused on work that they do not send text messages to their partner, and this can lead to misunderstandings and hurt, when the issue is not a lack of caring, but autistic monotropism – the tendency to focus on only one thing at a time.

One mother told us: 'He is in a very caring, loving relationship and at some point they will be intimate and that scares me. She's not on the spectrum and is very responsible. Both her mother and I have had family chats with them about protection and being careful – condoms, contraception – but it still scares me. They want to get married and have kids. He's afraid of cooking. How will he take care of the family?'

> **'Right now, he's not interested in a relationship but I worry he will end up continuing to be lonely ... we're working on it.'**

'People will come to me as an adult and say, "I want a girlfriend", but they have never really practised what reciprocal interaction with somebody is,' says Jodi Rodgers from Birds and Bees, a counselling service for people with disabilities. Rodgers, author of *Unique: What autism can teach us about difference, connection and belonging*, is a sexologist and special education teacher with thirty years' experience, focusing on relationships and sexual health. She says boys often have a special interest area through their teen years and that means they haven't had the same opportunities to be around women. This can present challenges on the dating scene. There can be other obstacles too: understanding what compromise looks like, especially if a partner does not share the same strong interests, and opportunities and access to meeting new people.

'Once people leave high school, then where do they actually go to meet people?' Rodgers acknowledges the ballooning number of dating apps that is now the most common way for people to meet. 'But people have to know how to have reciprocal communication through texting. Do they know what back and forth texting looks like?' She says the average number of dates a NT person will go on before they might enter a relationship is thirty-one. 'So, we've got to also talk to people about expectations in dating.' This includes rejection.

Setting expectations is also important because many ND people are vulnerable, and some jump in with the belief that their partner is 'the love of their life' very quickly. This is a period where young adults are also 'trialling people out, seeing what the good fit is and what rejection feels like. They're learning all of the social nuances. A lot of autistic people are not doing that in their high-school years or practising those skills in adulthood.' To overcome this, Rodgers role-plays and practises with clients. She says she might ask one question and will sometimes get a twenty-minute 'info dump' in response. 'And then I'll draw a social script or social autopsy. We'll think about perspective and point of view, which we know is very difficult for some autistic people.' What would someone be thinking after a twenty-minute Minecraft dump? 'It's really trying to teach people perspectives and point of view,' she says.

Rodgers understands the vulnerability felt by young adults. 'We're living in a world where we talk about people getting scammed all the time. And a lot of it is [happening] online.' Add to that the community expectation many feel to find a soulmate and it makes for a tricky highwire act. Relationships can hurt.

DATING TIPS FOR AUTISTIC YOUNG ADULTS

Jodi Rodgers from Birds and Bees regularly delivers workshops to people with a disability, with a focus on relationships, sexuality and sexual health. She recommends the following advice to prepare your ND teen for the dating scene.

- Does your teen have a friend and do they independently go out with that friend in the community? If you can't make and maintain a friendship, it's very hard to make and maintain a romantic relationship. Encourage your teen to develop friendships throughout their lives.
- Have realistic conversations about the reality of dating. This should include rejection. We all develop relationships differently. A 'hook-up' culture might mean many individuals are just looking for a short-term dalliance. Others want a long-term committed partnership. That means expectations can differ widely. Do you talk about this with your young people?
- Self-awareness, self-confidence and self-esteem are important. Does your teen know themselves? Are they confident and comfortable in themselves? These are important in dealing with vulnerability and understanding boundaries. They will also influence communication between partners.

HITTING THE ROAD

While many parents of young adults had concerns about their child being in a serious relationship, just as many mums and dads were worried about driving. 'I'm a mum of five children, three who are neurodiverse,' one mother told us. 'My motto to my kids is you all can do anything, maybe it may take us a little longer to achieve the goal but there is always a way around the hurdle. My seventeen-year-old daughter who is neurodiverse passed her driving test first time this year, something a lot of people never thought was possible, but she did it because there is always a way!'

DATING AND DRIVING

Jenny Gribbin is an occupational therapist who specialises in driving assessments; that means she determines if a medical condition or disability impacts on the ability of a person to drive safely. The national driver medical standards 'Assessing Fitness to Drive' sets out the considerations and medical criteria for safe driving. But here's what autistic drivers and those hoping to get a licence need to know. Those standards were updated with a section on 'other neurological conditions' now specifying 'autism' as a medical condition, and which might require a practical assessment. This is the same process for other conditions, including diabetes, epilepsy and eye disorders. Gribbin says research suggests that half the population with ND might be successful in gaining their driver's licence but it might take a ND person up to three times as long as others to learn to drive.

Cindi, who is autistic, was looking forward to the independence of learning to drive, but it took her a lot longer than many of her peers. Her instructor never taught her how to start the driving-school car: 'It was always running, including for her first test,' her mother says. She failed that test. 'The second time she had to start it and she couldn't. The instructor called to her as she walked to the car, "Just press the button three times, you'll be right." She couldn't get the car moving. She had no idea to put her foot on the brake or whatever it was to get the car to move, so she was stuck. The examiner then barked, "This is taking too long, you fail." And that was it, [she] never even left the carpark.' It took Cindi four tries over eight months to get her licence.

Gribbin says an occupational therapy 'potential to drive' assessment will usually end with one of four outcomes: a learner driver may not need any specialised support, and can continue through a mainstream service; they may need specialised driver training and occupational therapy; they might not be ready to drive yet – 'It's not a no, not ever, but they need to go away and work on some of those pre-driving skills first and develop more maturity'; or some people might have impairments, which means they are not able to drive or learn to drive.

While the guidelines are national, each state's licensing authority has a different testing process. For example, AustRoads has advised that licensed autistic drivers are not required to report their diagnosis to their state licensing authority if their symptoms are unlikely to affect their capacity to drive. Novice and learner autistic drivers are not required to report the diagnosis if their symptoms don't impact their ability to drive safely. But, Gribbin says, if they have any impairments, then those challenges could affect safe driving and cause problems with observation, processing and planning. It is important to get assessed, as this could mean the difference between being safe and having a crash.

While licensing processes might differ between states, Gribbin says they will generally involve the learner driver gaining a medical clearance from a GP, confirming they are medically stable with their diagnosis, and then report this to their state licensing authority; they may have a restriction on their licence. Occupational therapy driver assessors will assess the impact of the ND condition on driving and make recommendations about what supports are required to keep the driver safe. The complexity here means it's worth checking with your state licensing authority and your GP before submitting any applications for tests.

PART IV: THE FUTURE LOOKS BRIGHT

13. NDIS AND THE NEW LANDSCAPE

From a distance, the National Disability Insurance Scheme, or NDIS, looks a bit like a big lucky dip at a school fete. At first, it seems full of promise, having delivered funding to 650,000 Australians; the windfall for many means they can access a range of services to assist them to live independently. But often, like a lucky dip, it ends in disappointment; the deficit-based model means parents are forced to focus on a child's shortcomings – not their strengths – in a bid to boost their chance of winning the prize. Many parents also told us they had eschewed support because the application process required them to detail, over and over, what was 'wrong' with their child in a way that made them feel uneasy.

In those cases where NDIS funding is refused, parents are left exhausted, frustrated and even penniless. Many of the parents we spoke to criticised the scheme, claiming it is unfair, and in many cases stymied the future of their child who has just missed out on funding support because of arbitrary criteria.

That's not to decry the historic national disability system, introduced by former prime minister Julia Gillard in 2013 before a full nationwide roll-out in 2020. The NDIS has become part of our society's ecosystem and provides skills and support to help kids transition to school, find a job, participate in sport and leisure, and dozens of other competencies. The NDIS provides specialised support and therapy programs to deliver greater access for ND people to participate in their local community. In short, the aim is to level the playing field for everyone, and few could argue against the existence of the $30 billion scheme. It's *how* it has operated that continues to cause problems, especially when a parent or carer has only just received a diagnosis for their child.

In 2022 the concerns of parents and carers were acknowledged with a review of the NDIS, which identified the need to update the scheme. The review's recommendations, which aim to be both responsive and cost effective, have been welcomed by experts, practitioners and politicians. The hope is that old-fashioned labels that focus on levels or stages of disability will disappear from application forms and be replaced with criteria that focuses on a person's need for support.

Sydney mother Nicki Powell has an autistic son with ADHD and a general anxiety disorder. She says, 'The end goal is to get funding so you can support your child in areas they find challenging. Powell's business provides parents with coaching and support as they navigate applications to the NDIS. She recommends breaking the process down into small practical steps to reduce some of the anxiety that many parents experience when applying for help – and maybe even increase their chance of success.

Here's a snapshot of how many Australian families viewed the NDIS scheme as it stands:

- 'It has been a nightmare. I get teary just thinking about it and I feel overwhelmed by it. I feel like they have not

listened when I have requested increases in his funding. They do not understand how his diagnosis impacts other areas of his life, such as his body and how it functions. They do not understand the impact it has on the family.'
- 'Dealing with the NDIS is like being in a financially abusive relationship that you simply cannot afford to leave. Dealing with them is, at its core, trauma-inducing.'
- 'It is so exhausting to navigate. It's like they want to wear you down and make you stop trying. You have to push every step of the way. I was ringing weekly to get into any spare spot at about eight different child psychologists, then once on the NDIS it took me months to find placement with therapists. There is the constant worry that if your child improves that your funding will be cut, but it's that actual support which is seeing them improve, and if you take it away they may regress.'
- 'NDIS has provided our son with great resources but the pathway there was horrific. To succeed in accessing funding they first put you through a process whereby your child is described in detail as the sum of all their deficits. It breaks them down into a list of negative attributes that makes them sound like a drain on society. Then, and only then, they give you the resources the kids need to have equity in the health system.'
- 'It's traumatising, time consuming, expensive and completely dehumanising.'
- 'Brutal. Traumatic. Every year is a fight. Goal for NDIS is always to "heal" our son with as little money as possible.'

One of the issues at the heart of the unrest is the list of the conditions that are eligible for funding under the NDIS – and specifically what is missing from that list. One of those is ADHD, despite it being so common and debilitating for many families. That even led some parents to consider returning to a doctor in the hope that if they added another diagnosis to their child's chart, then ADHD might be addressed as part of it. As one parent told us: 'He is not eligible due to his diagnosis. It has been suggested we should seek an additional diagnosis of autism just to get some funding for social counselling with a psychologist, even though we don't believe this fits our boy.' Other families had a similar experience: 'I'm actually a support coordinator and find it really hard that ADHD isn't included, we missed the boat for early intervention due to school not really giving me the full picture with how much she was struggling.'

> **'ADHD is not funded and dyslexia is considered an issue for schools to deal with, leading to extraordinary costs for our family.'**

The picture painted by respondents to our survey showed, with startling clarity, the heartache that now begins with the application form. 'You have to beg to get help and even then, they expect you to jump through hoops while knitting a sweater. What they require for reports seems to change by the day, and they will deny you funding for the smallest things, like wording something wrong.' Others agreed that the paperwork was difficult to understand. 'I am well educated and if it wasn't for a fantastic paediatrician who walked me through how to apply, I would have got it wrong. Once we were set up it has been really good and made such a difference.'

Those who stuck with it and even demanded reviews of their application were often relieved they did – because it led to support and a funding package. 'It's been great – once we were approved, we had very supportive plans. It's paid for a lot of therapies we otherwise couldn't afford,' says one parent.

'Initially it was excruciating,' another parent agreed. 'Rewriting goals. Endless meetings. The stress of it was a factor in the end of our marriage. Now, it is less difficult to navigate; we have sufficient funding for supports.'

The difficulty of navigating the system was mentioned on multiple occasions. One mother told us, 'I am really grateful that the NDIS exists and that my kids can get support I could not otherwise afford. I have left two planning meetings in tears due to the way I have been spoken to, though. My daughter's plan is woeful and it frustrates me that because she masks outside the home she gets much less support than she needs.'

Inconsistencies abound too – where one family might get almost double what another family receive despite having made a similar application. 'Different people with similar autism levels get vastly different funding depending on who they got reports from,' one parent complained. 'We got $15,000 per year, but a friend with a girl – very similar and same age – got $30,000 per year.'

Independent experts and NDIS providers told us this usually comes down to individual NDIS planners seeing the applicant's challenges differently. 'I think it depends who you get on the day of your assessment – I know people who have breezed through with little documentation,' one parent said.

> 'I am grateful for the NDIS. Prior to it we neglected our mortgage and invested thousands into early intervention. That said, it is a deficit-based system and is an extremely traumatising process to endure.'

And, of course, families who live in regional areas are disadvantaged, with delays in getting a diagnosis and accessing expert health therapy once a package is approved, both of which are impacted by long waiting lists. 'We live in regional Queensland. Accessing face-to-face sessions for therapy means massive waiting lists – three years and still waiting. While we have funding for a support worker, we are unable to source someone to provide the service.' Other regional families acknowledge their expenses are often higher as they have to travel further for support. 'Regional kids do not receive equitable service delivery because of the amount of travel we pay from our child's package.'

Many of the issues parents raised during our research were also raised in the review of the NDIS, led by Professor Bruce Bonyhady AM and Lisa Paul AO PSM. The report was delivered in late 2023 and made twenty-six recommendations, involving 139 supporting actions. This included that access be based on level of impairment and not strictly and only on a medical diagnosis. While this is supported by families, doctors, therapists and academics, the current system still operates on labels. For example, most autistic people are eligible for funding, unless it's 'low-level'. People with ADHD are not supported through NDIS. The review also gave credibility to these concerns around inequity, saying some participants could automatically access the system because of a diagnosis, but not the support they required. 'A focus on functional impairment will enable multiple disabilities to be considered – which when taken together, result in significant functional impairment,' the review said.

Several families, after being rejected by NDIS, have appealed the decision, and taken their case to the courts, particularly the Administrative Appeals Tribunal (AAT), with mixed success.

'It's an absolute nightmare,' one parent said. 'Have had to go to AAT and fight every step of the way and still don't have enough funding because apparently caring for a nine-year-old like she's two is normal.' And: 'I'd rather be grinding my face on concrete. I've been to the AAT to get very basic needs met for my son, only to be told "he wasn't disabled enough". The case was really hard, emotionally, to go through, given I have ADHD myself. The representative from the National Disability Insurance Agency (NDIA) actually asked me seriously what "self-care skills" were.'

Universal support for the NDIS to change focus and target 'functional capacity' rather than relying on a strict diagnosis will lead to change over the next five years. According to experts, moving forward, the label given in a diagnosis will largely be irrelevant when it comes to accessing NDIS support; the focus will move to the assistance required for a person to be able to function fully.

While all this points to the NDIS changing (and no doubt contracting), it could take several years. Professor Andrew Whitehouse is widely sought by governments to provide advice around disability supports, the NDIS, and the education system. He says it is highly unlikely that a medical diagnosis will confer eligibility for NDIS support within five years, and functional impairment – across the board – was seen as a fairer way to access help. 'It will be based on the needs of a particular person. I think it will be also true that there will be a range of other systems that will have greater investment in them,' he says. State-run early childhood development systems, for example, as well as the broader education system would be a focus of reform. 'For me, I think the education system is just about the most important frontier to conquer in how we can have happy, healthy kids turned into happy, healthy adults,' Whitehouse says. This is a highwire act, because as the NDIS is constricted by costs, the education system needs commensurate investment to provide support. The end product will mean fewer people will access NDIS, but it will be focused on those who need the most support.

Whitehouse has also been appointed to the National School Resourcing Board, which oversees school funding models. He makes no secret of his views about the absence of ND training for teachers: 'Teaching courses do not have a major component of teaching around neurodivergence and neuro-affirming education, when in their first year of teaching [in classrooms] they will encounter ND children and that will be taking up a significant amount of their time.' Whitehouse says teachers are seeking the knowledge and the 'notion that we can't be teaching this because there's no space in the curriculum is madness'.

NAVIGATING THE SYSTEM

So, how can a family today navigate the NDIS and increase their chances of support? What do they need to do? And what evidence should they gather?

Nicki Powell says she wishes she had a travel guide to negotiate the journey to support when her son was first diagnosed. 'There's a lot of grief and a lot of different emotions one has when faced with a diagnosis, because it's very unknown,' she says. Powell now helps other families on that support journey, which can start when a child is any age. Indeed, up until the age of six, an official diagnosis is not required to access NDIS support – although there are requirements to show evidence of developmental delays, or the need for a multidisciplinary team to support a child. From the age of six, however, a diagnosis is required from a paediatrician or multidisciplinary team if the child is under eighteen, and usually a psychiatrist if the applicant is an adult.

If a child is aged under nine years, parents or carers seeking NDIS support need to lodge an application with local organisations in their community, known as early childhood partners. The NDIS website provides information on how to connect with early childhood partners and local area coordinators. The application, which discusses the child and their diagnosis, if they have one, can be done verbally or via a form. Once that form is completed, the applicant is usually asked to provide supporting evidence, which will then lead to a meeting to discuss eligibility. If successful, a further planning meeting will discuss goals and a pathway forward for the applicant child.

Let's pause here, because those words 'supporting evidence' are crucial. What do you need to gather and take to that meeting which will help support your case?

It's worth remembering this: the NDIS considers the functional capacity of a child, or applicant, in six key areas:

1. Mobility
2. Communication
3. Social Interaction
4. Self-management
5. Learning
6. Self-care

It's important to provide documentation that might support a child's challenges in those specific areas. Powell suggests three pieces of evidence, including any professional reports, a family impact statement and a letter from the child's teacher.

Professional reports are likely to be sourced from a speech pathologist, an occupational therapist or a paediatrician the child has seen. The family impact statement might simply be a diary of your family's day, which could illustrate the difficulty in leaving the house in time because of your child's challenges, identify developmental delays or describe the amount of support they need to move through the day. It's worth doing this to show the different routines on both a school day and a weekend day, and to highlight the daily support a child might need through their waking hours. The third piece of evidence Powell suggests is a letter or bullet-point note from a teacher, who sees the child during class or in the playground. This piece of evidence underpins the discussion in earlier chapters and the need for families to develop a good relationship with their child's teacher, and for teachers to understand they might provide the gateway for families to receive support. Teachers are able to see children, working next to peers, for hours each day – and whether through observation or assessment, they can provide valuable information.

The meeting to discuss eligibility and a path forward will include discussion around the goals you have for your child. It might be worth thinking of those in terms of the six functional capacities the NDIS considers, as outlined on the previous page. Powell suggests six or seven goals, in total, is ideal. They can be broad, from transitioning to school or increasing social skills through teamwork. Two typical supports on offer through the NDIS are occupational therapy and speech therapy. Our research indicated that while psychological services were available, many families found it harder to get funding for these.

That said, there is a wide landscape of other offerings that can truly make a difference in other ways. For example, Powell's son loves a Dungeons & Dragons course that helps him learn communication and social skills. Other suggestions run from boxing classes to art therapy to exercise physiology, and almost everything in between – as long as it helps your child reach their goals. Of course, there are other commonsense rules: the activities need to be related to the disability, provide value for money, be reasonable and effective.

Consider the supports you want for your child that are going to have the biggest benefit for them. Powell says it's important to keep the end goal in mind because the discussions around your child can be heartbreaking; the NDIS operates under a deficit model that focuses on what your child *can't* do, instead of what they *can* do. After the meeting the family will later be informed about the financial package available to them. It will also be directed into different 'buckets' based on the goals outlined in the meeting.

In our experience, the bigger packages are usually given to younger children; a recognition, perhaps, of the value of early intervention. But whatever plan is offered, there are usually three choices in how it is managed: firstly, it can be managed by the NDIA, which means you can only use NDIS-registered providers; secondly, it can be managed by a partner planner who will deal with all the service providers; or finally, it can be self-managed, which provides more autonomy in terms of the professionals who are on the child's team. In this case, the services are paid upfront and then claimed back.

A note here: this explanation is for children aged from birth to nine years of age. If the applicant is over nine (and up to sixty-five), a local area coordinator, not an early childhood partner, manages the initial assessment. More questions and forms are part of the process for an older child, although the process is similar.

A second note: the NDIS does not provide funds to schools for individualised education or learning programs that can be provided by the school sector. That money is sourced separately by schools, based on disabilities within the student body. While some schools in some states will allow NDIS-funded therapists onto school grounds, others do not. The benefit is that a family can provide assistance specific to their child through their own package and this therapy can occur on-site during school hours. Because a child can be exhausted by the time the school bell rings at the end of the day, it can be futile to then take them to a long list of therapy appointments. Therapy at school is aimed at making it easier for the child, not harder for others.

Taken as a big picture, NDIS is a smart and revolutionary policy that helps hundreds of thousands of families each year. 'It's been our lifesaver,' one family said. But inconsistencies and hurdles in the system can make it difficult. For example, families with similar challenges should not end up with wildly different packages. The review process should be made simpler – remember you are entitled to a review, but it means the package can also be adjusted downwards. Waiting lists, particularly in rural areas, can be long and tortuous and need to be addressed. Too many families are travelling long distances just to get an appointment, leaving siblings and one parent hundreds of kilometres away. The reliance on an official diagnosis and not the functional challenge a child has also needs to be addressed; a point made by the NDIS review, which suggested a five-year transition to its recommended changes. And the system needs to be able to provide in a better way for those children who camouflage or mask their condition.

Over time, with the goodwill of those who dispense the funds and those who seek support, many of these issues will be resolved. But parents applying for support in the meantime will still have to face these challenges. It's worth re-emphasising for these families the advice of NDIS sherpa Nicki Powell: 'Remember that end goal – support for your child. Just remember the end goal.'

TIPS FOR TACKLING NDIS FUNDING APPLICATIONS

Nicki Powell offers the following tips to parents who are starting their NDIS journey:

- Don't think you need to do this alone. The NDIS, or partner organisations, can offer support. Find your local support networks and make an appointment to see them.
- Know the six 'functional domains' the NDIS considers when assessing your application: mobility, communication, social interaction, self-management, learning and self-care.
- Gather support material. Ensure reports and letters specify the disability, its permanency, and how it impacts on your child's daily life. Evidence can include family impact statements, a specialist or therapist report and a report by a teacher.
- Parents frequently reported that the NDIS deficit model can be challenging. Don't lose sight of the goal – more support for your child.
- The NDIS process does not define your child. It simply offers your child a means of support.

14. RESEARCH AND THE WAY AHEAD

MOTHER, MEDICO AND RESEARCHER DR Mandira Hiremath is a Victorian paediatrician, specialising in autism assessments. She admits how 'difficult' it was for her and her husband when the first of their two autistic children was diagnosed. 'Even despite my training, when we were faced with the diagnosis, it hit us hard,' she said. They started treating their young son differently, with kid gloves. But a month later, she thought, 'hang on a minute, this is the same kid' – 'It hit home that he's still that really cool kid who knows every truck name, and he's amazing at maths.' She started to wonder why she was treating him like he had a lifelong illness. 'It really put that theory into practice for me and really reframed how I talk to families now. I tell them that diagnosis is just a mini-handbook to help them understand their child better.' When a challenge arises, they can draw on that knowledge to be the best possible parent and allow their child to become the little human they want to be. Later, Hiremath's younger daughter was diagnosed with autism. Her husband has ADHD, and she reveals this with pride.

Hiremath's home experience also makes it easier for her to answer questions posed by parents whose children are diagnosed with a neurodivergence. She says the first question parents usually ask relates to how they can help their child; the second revolves around the possibility of their child 'growing out' of autism or being able to live a 'normal' life. 'In terms of growing out, I say "no" this is who your child is. This is how their brain works. But there will be some days when you don't see the spectrum because they're cruising along.' More likely, the challenges will come in transitioning from primary to secondary school, when starting a job, or beginning a relationship.

How does she answer the question about their child living a life like their peers?

It depends on any co-occurring conditions, but she says her answer is usually, 'Yes, they will find a job and if you support them to follow those passion areas and find their tribe, they're going to be super happy with their lives.'

Creating a pathway for ND kids into adulthood, and the skills needed to do that, are at the vanguard of Australian research into autism. From gold star national guidelines for diagnosis and the use of technology in delivering assessments and care, to early intervention and hopes of remodelling the education system – the focus on research has turned the corner away from the 'cause' of the condition, to smoothing the obstacles strewn on the path that neurodivergent people are likely to travel.

GENETICS AND BIOLOGY

Let's just take a rest on that path, briefly, to clarify what we know about the causes of autism before pointing to what lies ahead. Professor Adam Guastella from the Brain and Mind Centre at the University of Sydney says genetics and biology play a significant role in both autism and ADHD. He says historical research and clinical efforts have been 'siloed' with little effort investigating both conditions. Now that it is recognised that a person could have both, there is a 'growing awareness that most of the factors that are predictive of autism are also predictive of ADHD and other developmental conditions'.

Professor of Autism at the Telethon Kids Institute and the University of Western Australia Andrew Whitehouse says the role played by genetic differences has been well-established for many years and came from molecular genetic studies. 'The genes certainly change the way that the brain develops. It develops differently to what we typically expect,' he says. But Whitehouse, like other experts, says there is no one cause for why people show autistic behaviours. 'If you have ten people with a diagnosis of autism in a room you will almost certainly have ten different biological ways in which that person has come to show the behaviours we call autism.'

Clinical psychologist Dr Jessica Paynter is an associate professor at Griffith University in Queensland and a former president of the Australasian Society for Autism Research. She says a 'constellation of variables' need to interact to cause autism. For example, an extremely premature infant has a higher probability of being autistic than another infant. Paynter has been involved in one longitudinal study, which showed about ten per cent of children who were born before twenty-six weeks' gestation went on to meet the criteria for an autism diagnosis at the age of four. This matched the number of parents in our survey who said their ND child had been born prematurely. But many other factors could play a role, too, revealing the complexity around discussion of causes and risks. Scientists and researchers also point to the possible role of toxin exposure, the age of a child's parents at birth, the role a virus might play during pregnancy, or taking legal, but not-recommended, medications or illegal drugs. The relationship between the gut and autism continues to be explored.

Any role played by vaccines in contributing to autism has been dismissed categorically by every expert we interviewed. Guastella also makes this point: discussion on causes relates to those who have a diagnosis; many people are not diagnosed with autism or ADHD but still might exhibit the same behaviours. He says a range of social factors – including access to assessment, economics and even geography – could determine whether people were diagnosed or not.

'But there is no single cause,' Paynter confirms, 'and I think people would agree that we're not going to find a single cause now.'

LEADING THE WAY

The ND community is leading the way in putting ND people on an equal playing field. The medical model – involving diagnosis and assessments based on meeting certain criteria – is no longer seen as an acceptable approach. The efforts of the ND community have helped sway research energies and also reflects a broader view, across science and research, that autism should be seen as a difference, not a disorder. Indeed, some voices in the autistic community eschew the word 'disability', although Whitehouse cautions against this. 'I think we also have to be really clear that when we talk about autism as a difference – as we should – that we don't overlook the fact that these differences can create disabilities as well. There's a very significant proportion of kids who are not able to talk, and who have significant intellectual disability,' he says. 'These kids can be treasured for who they are, with all of their amazing personality and characteristics and neurodivergence. But we also must identify and support them in the disability they experience in the world in which they're born. I don't think that we can talk just about difference, we also have to talk about disability – otherwise these people's existence is simply going to be sugar-coated over.'

While big advances have been made in detecting and diagnosing autism, including non-binding recommended national guidelines, recent research is directed at 'real life outcomes and making things better for autistic people', Paynter says. 'Autistic people are actually setting the research priorities and addressing the issues that matter to them.' In addition to changing the focus, autistic researchers are also guiding and informing the way data is interpreted and safeguarding the way information is used.

Professor of Speech Pathology at Griffith University David Trembath says the involvement and leadership of the ND community is strongly influencing the approach to research: 'From the design, the questions that are asked, methods or approaches used, how we collect and then interpret information. And most importantly, what comes out of it: the recommendations,' he says. 'It's more fun. It's more interesting. It's more exciting, and it's better.'

Autistic academic Leia Greenslade says a good chunk of the research into ND people is now being led by ND researchers. 'I think we are seeing a split between the old method of non-ND researchers studying ND people (and often coming up with outrageously ableist research questions, methods and findings) and a new wave of ND researchers who are doing a much better job of centring ND needs throughout the whole process,' Greenslade said. 'I probably get an email from a ND student wanting to do research on their communities every couple of weeks. Currently, I have two PhD students, both ND themselves, studying how best to support ND students in Outside School Hours Care (OSHC) in Australia, and the other student is exploring how ND people make sense of their identities.' Across the board, the role played by ND researchers and scientists, leading and co-leading projects, is now considered crucial.

This push for research to focus on supports and not causes is a recommendation made repeatedly by experts over recent years, including in the formal review of the NDIS, which currently demands a diagnosis and prohibits assistance for some conditions, such as ADHD. Overwhelmingly, from diagnosis to funding, the advice is that the medical model should give way to best practice in addressing those obstacles that might prevent a neurodivergent person from reaching their full potential. Trembath says a focus on support was a 'fundamental message' of updated national guidelines around diagnosis and assessment.

'The diagnosis is helpful in some ways, in some places and cases and for some people.' But focusing on support needs could materially help those who require it, daily. Assessing functioning capabilities and projecting a picture of where a person could be are likely to take centrestage in coming years. 'Medical evaluation and diagnosis should absolutely be part of the picture, but it shouldn't be the key driver behind decision-making,' Trembath says.

A move away from diagnosis might certainly unlock support for some – partly because some conditions, like ADHD, are now not eligible for funding under the NDIS. This doesn't mean that it will become eligible, but that the NDIS will focus on the support someone requires, and not the diagnosis they have been given. Guastella says the system has been too diagnostically driven 'in terms of which children get support and which children don't'. This had led to huge waiting lists for diagnosis, and then a queue to access services. Some providers are also over-charging as a result, and it means children are not getting support as early as they could.

Experts believe the new focus of addressing needs has to use technology, involve multi-disciplinary levels of support – including teacher education – and envelop childcare settings and the school environment. 'I think it's a real shift ... to provide universal supports and provide some targeted supports to kids in their everyday settings,' Guastella says.

What excites Whitehouse is that it turns the corner on research that 'was running into dead ends'. He says, 'There is focus on the human potential that every child, no matter how they're born, is beautiful. Rather than getting tangled up in knots about the genetics, we are focusing on that child and how we can actually help them be who they want to be.'

NEW RESEARCH DIRECTIONS

As research into the causes of neurodivergence is declining, it is being replaced with studies that are trying to pinpoint the best support needed within the ND community. Massive longitudinal studies are underway overseas, including in the US and the UK, which will take many years to assess. Much of the exciting Australian research, though, is being conducted on evidence-based pathways to helping children early. Here are a couple of examples, which provide hope for ND children and their families.

The Inklings Program was developed over a twenty-year

period by an international team of researchers in the UK and Australia. This program – directed at children aged six to eighteen months – is considered a game-changer. It has been rolled out across Western Australia and was implemented in South Australia in 2024, after clinical studies involving fifty-four babies in the UK and more than 100 babies in Australia (aged between nine and fourteen months) showed stunning results. Children who received early intervention were two-thirds less likely to later reach the criteria for an autism diagnosis. In Australia, children are earmarked for the program if they have a sibling with autism or who have early behavioural signs of autism.

The study, led by Professor Whitehouse and the Perth-based Telethon Kids Institute, included Western Australia's Child and Adolescent Health Service, La Trobe University, the University of Western Australia and the University of Manchester. Both low-cost and family-based, the Inklings Program helps parents understand what their baby might be thinking and feeling, and how to follow their cues and responses. Babies are born able to communicate, but those social and communication skills can develop differently to what we might expect. For example, differences might be in how they respond to their name or an instruction, how they play or their eye gaze.

The program teaches parents and carers how to respond to their child's way of communicating before the age of three, when autism can typically be diagnosed. Instead of trying to change developmental differences, this program – using videos of the parents and children playing – provides feedback on the way the child is communicating and how parents could respond. Whitehouse says the program has massive potential, given that fifty-three per cent of all children on the NDIS now have a diagnosis of autism. 'What it means is the child learns in a way that is best for them, rather than the way that's best for us, and that supports their development so much more,' he says.

The work of Associate Professor Josephine Barbaro from the La Trobe University's Olga Tennison Autism Research Centre has also conducted world-first research into early screening. She developed a tool that allows a child to be diagnosed much earlier for autism, thereby improving developmental outcomes and early access to support and therapy.

Sydney University also has several projects underway. One of these has shown that people with ND conditions are at much higher risk of serious mental health concerns and find it harder to access support. Professor Guastella, along with postdoctoral research fellow Kelsie Boulton and Associate Professor Natalie Silove, assessed mental health symptoms in children attending their first assessment. Using the Sydney Child Neurodevelopment Research Registry, they found that about half of the children showed 'clinical levels of mental heath symptoms'. This increased to seventy per cent for children with co-occurring or multiple diagnoses.

The study involved 232 families who were asked about their child's mental health when they first attended a broader neurodevelopmental assessment. Guastella says the reasons why those presenting with ND conditions have higher mental health concerns are complex and could relate to social factors, such as discrimination, peer rejection and exclusion, as well as family separation and conflict or social isolation, among others. He says ND conditions could also be associated with attention difficulties, impulsivity, stress and emotional regulation.

The takeaway here is that mental health care should be central to the care of those with ND conditions and delivered as early as possible. The barriers to access are broad, with Guastella's team nominating a lack of training in mental health and incorrect beliefs by professionals that ND people might be too complex to respond to supports, unwieldy government structures and referral pathways for funding and services, stigma and discrimination, and access issues. 'A failure to provide mental health supports when symptoms first develop results in more acute and chronic issues,' the team wrote in a 2023 article for *The Conversation*. ND people are more likely to present at acute mental health facilities and emergency services, and be admitted for complex mental health problems. 'Sadly, autistic people also have a tenfold higher risk of suicide, compared to people without ND conditions. That's why this study is important.'

Guastella says ongoing research is broad and also includes using technology to break down siloed information. For example, in one project, data is being collected at clinics and education services to track children over time and provide feedback. Instead of data being stored in filing cabinets or kept on discrete servers, it is put into an integrated research database which allows researchers to anonymously track the journey of children as they enter clinical services, and ties that to support needs and educational outcomes. 'It becomes an opportunity for families to get access to research and to be involved in understanding outcomes for children in rural and remote areas, and then we can build digital tools to support those children as well,' he says. 'It means that our findings and our work directly translate into what's happening in clinical practice on a daily basis.'

Back in Victoria, research is underway into teaching neurodiversity in primary school. Dr Hiremath's PhD in this field has a backstory, which started with a family visit to the

US in 2023. One of her nieces is autistic and has an intellectual disability. 'She entered into a mainstream school, and she got severely bullied and discriminated against and just felt really isolated' Hiremath says. 'So, her mum became a really big advocate for her and instituted an education program for all primary school students about neurodiversity.' This included a buddy system between neurodiverse children and NT children to help form friendships and try and reduce the instances of bullying. In short, the outcome was successful and prompted Hiremath to focus on what neurodiversity education programs existed in Australia. She found some for teens and parents, relating to health, but none for younger students. Her PhD, undertaken at Monash University, looks at providing education about neurodiversity within primary schools, 'and what that might look like to all primary school students', she says.

In our own research, parents found NT children with an understanding of diversity could be the gold nugget in school friendships; those who had been taught by their parents to value difference were able to materially change the school days of some ND students who were struggling. Hiremath's work – including co-designing a program with schools, health professionals, parents and students – is expected to begin in mid-2025 with a limited in-school pilot program. This would be used to compare how specific neurodiversity education might change the primary school environment in terms of how students and teachers saw difference. Hiremath's work is personal as much as professional. 'I haven't told anybody in my kids' school apart from the teachers that my children are on the spectrum and that's because of the stigma and the fear of judgement. I want children to be able to go into school, be themselves, find their tribes, and that'll only happen if other children feel confident in that environment, and parents also feel confident in that environment. For me, this is a big step in contributing to that changing world.'

THE FUTURE LOOKS BRIGHT

Certainly, the breadth of research being undertaken into developing support for the ND community signals a new beginning. Many senior management courses are now focusing on neurodiversity on boards and in leadership teams. Some experts are full of optimism, saying neurodiversity is now tracking the same path that sexual and gender identification has paved in recent years. 'I think this is the next wave coming,' one says.

But there's still a long way to go. Dr Catherine Franklin, psychiatrist, researcher and director of the Mater Intellectual Disability and Autism Service in Brisbane says there is much work to do on understanding the environment, as much as the person, in forging better outcomes for autistic children. 'The problem we have now is a thing called diagnostic overshadowing – if an autistic person turns up at a mental health service and has depression and is suicidal, they can be told "we don't do autism" here or "it's probably just your autism". And that happens every day.' Likewise, she's had instances of people who have been coughing up blood and being told it is 'their autism or their behaviour', which reveals a fundamental lack of understanding, including from some GPs. Franklin says the health system and governments will have to disrupt their operations to better meet the demands of ND people seeking support. 'Their opinion remains that autistic people should access mainstream services and should be able to, but they can't get help from mainstream services. So, it's a really difficult position.'

Franklin says more than ninety per cent of autism research involves children, highlighting a dearth of information about adults. This suggests that the mental health of autistic adults might not be getting the attention it should, and reflects the views of Assistant Minister for Autism in South Australia Emily Bourke. Her appointment to the new role – the first of its type we could find – followed a series of community forums by the Labor Party in the lead-up to the state's 2022 election. 'Autism just kept coming up in all of those forums,' Bourke says. Statistics she's found around autism are alarming: if you are autistic you are half as likely to finish Year 10, three times more likely to be unemployed and those who get to the age of fifty are considered 'an old autistic'.

Bourke worries that most people know the word 'autism' but don't have any deeper knowledge. She is particularly concerned about the gap in focus on older people, who might be undiagnosed autistic. 'There's been a lot of focus on the younger generations and even my demographic, the forty-year-old,' she says. That's partly driven by the knowledge of the role played by genetics, so when a child is diagnosed, often a parent will also choose to be diagnosed. She says familial links in autism mean that parents are becoming a focus for diagnosis, but not necessarily grandparents. 'We've got people potentially going into aged care or support earlier than they necessarily need to be, because there's not the understanding that they might be autistic,' she says.

Franklin provides a reminder that autism has had a long and winding history. While it was first lumped in with schizophrenia, institutionalisation was later considered an answer to many of the articulated problems. Then 'autism' was divided into stages or types, and the term Asperger's was introduced. Now that word is no longer used widely (although some families with an autistic child prefer its use).

'It's been an interesting journey,' Franklin says. 'And like many things, the pendulum swings on a global level.' But for a long time, society didn't want to know about it. Now, with widespread recognition, increased understanding and serious research, the road looks wide open.

RESOURCES: FOR PARENTS

AUTISM AND ADHD ORGANISATIONS AND EXPERTS

Amaze provides a range of services in advocacy and education for autistic individuals, including workshops, training and resources on topics such as the NDIS, mental health, education and employment. Amaze offers Australia's first national autism helpline: Autism Connect. (www.amaze.org.au)

DivergAntz Collective is a group of neuro-affirming professionals committed to improving the diagnosis journey. They offer services such as therapy and cognitive assessment, as well as professional courses, skills training and resources. (www.divergantz.com.au)

Minds & Hearts is a clinic specialising in neurodevelopmental disorders, including autism, ADHD and learning difficulties, as well as attachment issues and emotion regulation challenges. Run by Dr Wesley Turner and Dr David Zimmerman, their goal is to work with individuals and families to discover and build self-understanding. (www.mindsandhearts.net)

RESOURCES: FOR PARENTS

Yellow Ladybugs is an autistic-led charity dedicated to the happiness and success of autistic girls, women and gender diverse individuals. They provide neuro-affirming education, resources and safe connection opportunities while advocating for the rights of their community. (www.yellowladybugs.com.au)

Jodi Rodgers is a qualified sexologist, counsellor and special education teacher and the relationship specialist on *Love on the Spectrum: Australia*. She set up Birds and Bees to provide parents and educators with practical tools and resources for teaching children about sexuality in a positive and age-appropriate manner. (www.birdsandbees.com.au)

Andrew Whitehouse is the Professor of Autism Research and Director of CliniKids at the Telethon Health Institute. CliniKids is a network of clinical centres for children with neurodevelopmental differences that embeds clinical trials within everyday community practice. He also presents a video series called '60 Second Silence' and regularly advises government on policy relating to autistic children. (www.clinikids.telethonkids.org.au/)

Bronwyn Sutton is a speech pathologist and educator who works with autistic children and their families. She provides neurodiversity affirming coaching sessions to parents to help them better communicate and support their child.

Kristy Forbes is an autism advocate, consultant and educator based in Australia. She provides support for individuals and families living with autism and related conditions, offering consultancy services, resources and workshops. (www.kristyforbes.com.au)

Michelle Garnett is a clinical psychologist specialising in autism. Alongside Professor Tony Attwood she co-founded Attwood & Garnett Events, to enhance autism awareness and understanding. (www.attwoodandgarnettevents.com)

Nicki Powell is an educator who provides a consultancy to help parents find appropriate support services for diagnosing their child and guiding them through the process of accessing NDIS funding, as well as assisting with kids transitioning from home to preschool and into primary school. (www.nickipowell.com.au)

Ross Greene is a clinical psychologist and originator of the Collaborative and Proactive Solutions (CPS) Model (www.cpsconnection.com), a tool to help solve problems that are causing concerning behaviour in children. (www.drrossgreene.com)

Russell Barkley is a leading expert on ADHD and executive functioning disorders. His website holds a wealth of information on ADHD diagnosis, treatment and management strategies for individuals, families and professionals. (www.russellbarkley.org)

Tony Attwood is a leading voice in neurodiversity currently serving as an adjunct professor at Griffith University. He co-founded Attwood & Garnett Events in 2019, which offers informative webcasts and online courses for parents of autistic children. (www.attwoodandgarnettevents.com)

PARENTING EXPERTS AND ORGANISATIONS

Casey Ehrlich is a social scientist, parenting coach and mindfulness practitioner. Her website offers resources and support for parents navigating challenges in raising children. (www.atpeaceparents.com)

Justin Coulson is a renowned parenting expert and author dedicated to helping families cultivate happiness and harmony in their homes. His website offers a wide range of resources, courses, webinars and podcasts focused on practical strategies for building strong family relationships. (www.happyfamilies.com.au)

Karen Young is an author and anxiety consultant. She is the mind behind Hey Sigmund, an online trove of research-driven insights and resources for understanding and improving mental health, anxiety and emotional wellbeing. (www.heysigmund.com)

Maggie Dent is a respected author, educator and parenting expert. Her websites provide a wealth of articles, webinars, courses and events to help parents and educators nurture children's wellbeing and development. (www.maggiedent.com; www.commonsenseparenting.com.au)

Mary Kaspar is the author of *The Popular Girls: Helping Your Daughter with Adolescent Power Struggles*. She also provides workshops for parents and students within school communities to help guide teenagers towards fostering healthy relationships. (www.drmarykaspar.com.au)

Mona Delahooke is a clinical psychologist specialising in childhood development and trauma-informed care. Her website offers resources and insights on promoting children's mental health and emotional wellbeing through compassionate and evidence-based approaches. (www.monadelahooke.com)

Naomi Fisher is a clinical psychologist specialising in child and adolescent mental health, offering therapy and support services for children, adolescents and families. Her website provides resources and insights on fostering emotional wellbeing and resilience in young people. (www.naomifisher.co.uk)

Rebecca Sparrow is a teen educator, the author of six books and the host of ABC's *Parental As Anything, Teens* podcast. She specialises in teaching tweens, teens and their parents about friendship: how to find friends, recognise healthy friendships, build robust relationships, avoid drama and navigate conflict. Her online webinars are watched by families around the world. Bec is also the co-founder of Books with Bec & Jane, online book clubs for kids, teens and adults. (www.rebeccasparrow.com)

Tosha Schore is an expert in attachment-based parenting. Parenting Boys Peacefully offers resources and guidance for parents seeking to nurture their sons with compassion and understanding, focusing on fostering emotional intelligence and healthy relationships. (www.parentingboyspeacefully.com)

FURTHER LEARNING AND ONLINE SUPPORT

Amazing Skills provides online and in-person small group classes that teach social skills and friendship skills to autistic kids and teens. (www.amazingskills.com.au)

Community Against Prejudice Towards Autistic People (CAPTAP) is a network aimed at creating and connecting a community of people who are passionate about reducing stigma and prejudice towards autistic people. (www.captapnetwork.wordpress.com)

RESOURCES: FOR PARENTS

eXceptional Learners is a website offering specialised educational resources and support for learners with exceptionalities, focusing on personalised learning experiences and fostering inclusivity in education. (www.xceptionallearners.com)

FreeSchool is a not-for-profit organisation offering academic assistance to high-school kids. If your child is struggling at school, or not attending school (for whatever reason) or if they just need some extra help, head to their website, click on their year level and subject and you'll find video tutorials by amazing teachers. (www.freeschool.org.au)

GingerCloud Foundation is a Brisbane-based organisation devoted to removing the barriers experienced by ND young people with autism, Down Syndrome, ADHD or learning and perceptual disabilities. They run a number of programs, including the Modified Rugby Program, Player2PlayerMentor Pathway, Disability Inclusion Leaders Program, as well as work experience opportunities. (www.gingercloud.org)

NewAccess is a confidential guided six-session mental health coaching program provided by Beyond Blue for people who are feeling stressed or overwhelmed about everyday life issues such as work, study, relationships, health or loneliness. (www.beyondblue.org.au/get-support/newaccess-mental-health-coaching)

PEERS® stands for Program for the Education and Enrichment of Relational Skills and offers a range of structured social skills intervention programs aimed at adolescents and young adults with social challenges. It teaches strategies to improve social interactions and relationship conversation skills, electronic communication, appropriate use of humour and dating etiquette. (www.semel.ucla.edu/peers)

Planet Puberty was created by Family Planning NSW in collaboration with adults with intellectual disabilities and autism, and parents and experts. Planet Puberty offers a comprehensive digital resource suite to help parents and carers support their child through puberty. (www.planetpuberty.org.au)

Positive Partnerships provides information to parents, carers and educators of school-aged autistic children. Their website is full of practical tools and resources, as well as a planning tool to help summarise a young person's strengths and support needs at home, at school and in the community. They also run workshops and online training aimed at strengthening partnerships between parents and teachers. (www.positivepartnerships.com.au)

Reframing Autism aims to create a world in which the autistic community is supported by families and allies. Their mission is to change the frame through which society views autism, so that autistic people can flourish. They have created a sample letter for parents to give to teachers and other people in their child's support network – 'Neurodiversity-affirming Language: A Letter to Your Child's Support Network'. (www.reframingautism.org.au)

Secret Agent Society offers a suite of espionage-themed resources that are an evidence-based, comprehensive and captivating solution to structured social and emotional learning for children aged eight to twelve years old. (www.secretagentsociety.com)

RESOURCES: FOR PARENTS

Sex Ed Rescue was founded by renowned sex educator Cath Hakanson. Sex Ed Rescue offers comprehensive resources and courses for sex education, focusing on empowering parents and educators to navigate difficult conversations with children effectively and to promote healthy attitudes towards sexuality. (www.sexedrescue.com)

Social Thinking is targeted at helping individuals with ADHD, autism or social communication disorders. Their online training programs help people understand themselves and others to better navigate the social world, foster relationships and improve performance at school, home and work. (www.socialthinking.com)

The BRAVE Program is an online program developed by The University of Queensland for the prevention and treatment of childhood and adolescent anxiety. It's free, and provides children and teenagers with ways to cope with their worries (www.brave4you.psy.uq.edu.au)

The Spectrum Pharmacist was created by pharmacist Yvette Anderson to share her professional knowledge and personal experiences to empower the parents of ND children. Her website provides useful fact sheets on medications, tried and tested tips, as well as relevant links and honest advice about advocating for your neurodivergent child. (www.thespectrumpharmacist.com.au)

OTHER USEFUL WEBSITES

- www.adhdaustralia.org.au
- www.autism.org.au
- www.dyslexiaassociation.org.au

- www.healthdirect.gov.au
- www.ndis.gov.au
- www.neurodiversityhub.org
- www.ninds.nih.gov
- www.theactgroup.com.au
- www.headspace.org.au
- www.raisingchildren.net.au

BOOKS, PODCASTS AND MEDIA

NON-FICTION
- *ADHD an A–Z: Figuring it Out Step by Step* by Leanne Maskell
- *A Different Way to Learn: Neurodiversity and Self-Directed Education* by Naomi Fisher
- *Can't Not Won't: A Story About a Child Who Couldn't Go to School* by Eliza Fricker
- *Friendly Facts: A Fun, Interactive Resource to Help Children Explore the Complexities of Friends and Friendship* by Margaret-Anne Carter and Josie Santomauro
- *It's Not a Bloody Trend: Understanding Life as an ADHD Adult* by Kat Brown
- *Kit and Arlo Find a Way: Teaching Consent to 8–12 Year Olds* by Ingrid Laguna
- *Making Friends: A Guide to Getting Along with People* by Andrew Matthews
- *Scattered Minds: The Origins and Healing of Attention Deficit Disorder* by Gabor Maté
- *Spectrum Women: Walking to the Beat of Autism* by Michelle Garnett

RESOURCES: FOR PARENTS

- *The Body Keeps the Score: Mind, Brain and Body in the Transformation of Trauma* by Bessel van der Kolk
- *The Explosive Child: A New Approach for Understanding and Parenting Easily Frustrated, Chronically Inflexible Children* by Ross W. Greene
- *The Out-of-Sync Child: Recognizing and Coping with Sensory Processing Differences* by Carol Stock Kranowitz
- *The Neurodivergent Friendly Workbook of DBT Skills* by Sonny Jane Wise
- *The Science of Making Friends: Helping Socially Challenged Teens and Young Adults* by Elizabeth A Laugeson
- *What Is Friendship? Games and Activities to Help Children to Understand Friendship* by Pamela Day
- *Wild Things: How We Learn to Read and What Can Happen If We Don't* by Sally Rippin
- *Yes, Your Kid: What Parents Need to Know About Today's Teens and Sex* by Debby Herbenick
- *Your Brain's Not Broken: Strategies for Navigating Your Emotions and Life with ADHD* by Tamara Rosier

PODCASTS
- *ANOMALOUS* with Em Rusciano
- *Distracted* with Kat Wilson and Jack Suddaby
- *Dr Ross Greene Podcast Series*
- *Exploring Neurodiversity* with Adina Levy from Play. Learn. Chat
- *Pop Culture Parenting Podcast* with Dr Billy Garvey and Nick McCormack
- *The Sue Larkey Podcast*
- *The Village Lantern Podcast*
- *Too Peas in a Podcast*

MEDIA

- 'Adult ADHD', SBS *Insight* (www.sbs.com.au/ondemand/watch/1865101891814)
- 'Consent for Kids', Blue Seat Studios (www.youtube.com/watch?v=h3nhM9UlJjc)
- 'SuperSoul Sessions: The Anatomy of Trust', Brené Brown (www.brenebrown.com/videos/anatomy-trust-video)
- 'Tea and Consent', Thames Valley Police (www.youtube.com/watch?v=pZwvrxVavnQ)
- 'Why everything you know about autism is wrong', TEDx Talks (www.youtube.com/watch?v=A1AUdaH-EPM)

REPORTS

- 'National Autism Indicators Report: Family Perspectives on Services and Supports', a US report that focuses on families and explores what families think about the services their family member on the spectrum is receiving and how well their own support needs are being met, Drexel University Autism Institute, 2021 (www.policyimpactproject.org/family-perspectives-on-services-and-supports).

RESOURCES: FOR EDUCATORS

AUTISM AND ADHD ORGANISATIONS AND EXPERTS

Allison Davies is a neurologic music therapist known for her expertise in utilising rhythm and music to support wellbeing and learning. Her website provides webinars, resources and insights on neurodevelopment and the therapeutic benefits of music for individuals of all ages. (www.allisondavies.com.au)

Billy Garvey is a dad, podcaster, author and paediatrician who is passionate about helping those who care for kids – parents, educators, sports coaches, family support workers – by advancing their ability to guide healthy child development and mental health. (www.guidinggrowingminds.com)

Jonelle Fraser is an autistic educator with over twenty-five years' experience in the education and disability sectors. Fraser supports teachers and parents in understanding and nurturing children's learning differences, offering training and tools to promote inclusive education. (www.auroralearning.com.au)

Seth Perler is a coach and educator specialising in supporting students with learning differences. His website offers resources, coaching services and guidance for students, parents and educators to help individuals navigate challenges related to executive function and academic success. (www.sethperler.com)

Sue Larkey is a qualified educator with extensive experience in special education. Her website offers courses and resources to help educators teach children on the autism spectrum. It focuses on increasing engagement, developing positive behaviour support programs and providing training. (www.suelarkey.com.au)

FURTHER LEARNING AND ONLINE SUPPORT

Amazing Things Happen! is a video appropriate for a primary school setting that explains and raises awareness of autism among non-autistic kids and adults. (www.youtube.com/@AmazingThingsProject)

Assessment of Skills & Unsolved Problems (ASUP) is an online tool devised by Lives in the Balance for educators to identify lagging skills and look at proactive solutions for solving learning problems. All the resources you need to implement the CPS Model can be found on the website. (www.livesinthebalance.org/cps-materials-paperwork/)

Chloé Hayden is an autistic and ADHD award-winning speaker, actor, author, content creator and disability rights advocate. She delivers presentations at seminars, webinars, conferences and schools to spread her message of 'Different, Not Less'. (www.chloehayden.com.au)

RESOURCES: FOR EDUCATORS

Emotion Sensation Feeling Wheel has been adapted by Lindsay Braman to help people learn to recognise and name their emotions. (www.lindsaybraman.com/emotion-sensation-feeling-wheel)

Lives in the Balance is a non-profit organisation that provides tools and resources for parents, educators and professionals interested in understanding and addressing behavioural challenges. The Collaborative and Proactive Solutions (CPS) Model aims to dramatically reduce discipline referrals and detentions by offering improved problem-solving techniques. (www.livesinthebalance.org)

NeuroWild is run by autistic and ADHD speech pathologist, illustrator, advocate and mother of neurodiverse children, Emily Hammond. Her page captures complex concepts in fun and easy to understand illustrations. (www.facebook.com/p/NeuroWild-100087870753308)

Students with Disability is an Australian Government Department of Education website with a range of data and resources for schools and families about Disability Standards for Education and understanding learning difficulties. (www.education.gov.au/swd)

Talking About Autism is a toolkit created by Amaze with guidelines for respectful and accurate reporting on autism and autistic people. (www.amaze.org.au/wp-content/uploads/2020/09/Talking-about-autism-a-media-resource.pdf)

The Socially Speaking Game was designed by Alison Schroeder to complement her book, *Socially Speaking*. The board game focuses on social interaction at home, school and in the community. Children can practise skills such as greetings, turn-taking, eye contact, listening, compliments and building friendships.

BOOKS

- *All About PDA: An Insight Into Pathological Demand Avoidance* by Kathy Hoopmann
- *Building Healthy Friendships: Teaching Friendship Skills to Young People* by Terry A. Beck
- *Friendly Kids, Friendly Classrooms: Teaching Social Skills and Confidence in the Classroom* by Helen McGrath and Shona Francey
- *Making & Keeping Friends: Ready-to-Use Lessons, Stories, and Activities for Building Relationships* by John J. Schmidt
- *Socially Speaking: A Pragmatic Social Skills Programme for Pupils with Mild to Moderate Learning Disabilities* by Alison Schroeder
- *The Educator's Experience of Pathological Demand Avoidance : An Illustrated Guide to Pathological Demand Avoidance and Learning* by Laura Kerbey
- *The Essential Manual for Asperger Syndrome (ASD) in the Classroom: What Every Teacher Needs to Know* by Kathy Hoopmann

RESOURCES: FOR ND KIDS AND TEENS

BOOKS FOR PRIMARY SCHOOLERS

BOOKS ON NEURODIVERSITY
- *All Dogs Have ADHD* by Kathy Hoopmann
- *All Cats Are on the Autism Spectrum* by Kathy Hoopmann
- *Come Over to My House* by Eliza Hull and Sally Rippin
- *Dyslexia is My Superpower (Most of the Time)* by Margaret Rooke
- *Gus the Asparagus* by Anne-Marie Finn and Kaylene Hobson
- *Love Me, Love My ADHD* by Chrissie Davies
- *Some Brains: A Book Celebrating Neurodiversity* by Nelly Thomas
- *Square Me, Round World: Stories of Growing up in a World Not Built for You* by Chelsea Luker
- *The Asperkid's (Secret) Book of Social Rules: The Handbook of (Not-So-Obvious) Social Guidelines for Tweens and Teens with Asperger Syndrome* by Jennifer Cook
- *The Brain Forest* by Sandhya Menon
- *The Rainbow Brain* by Sandhya Menon

BOOKS ON ANXIETY
- *All Birds Have Anxiety* by Kathy Hoopmann
- *But We're Not Lions!* by Karen Young
- *Dear You, Love From Your Brain* by Karen Young
- *Hey Awesome* by Karen Young
- *Hey Warrior* by Karen Young
- *Ups and Downs: A Book for Kids About Big Feelings* by Karen Young

NOVELS WITH ND MAIN CHARACTERS
- *Counting by 7s* by Holly Goldberg Sloan
- *Fish in a Tree* by Lynda Mullaly Hunt
- *Harriet Hound* by Kate Foster
- *Paws* by Kate Foster
- *The Bravest Word* by Kate Foster
- *The Unlikely Heroes Club* by Kate Foster
- *Third Time's a Charm* by Kate Foster

BOOKS FOR HIGH SCHOOLERS

NON-FICTION
- *A Good Friend: How to Make One, How to Be One* by Ron Herron and Val J. Peter
- *Different, Not Less: A Neurodivergent's Guide to Embracing Your True Self and Finding Your Happily Ever After* by Chloé Hayden
- *Love & Autism* by Kay Kerr

RESOURCES: FOR ND KIDS AND TEENS

- *Socially Curious and Curiously Social: A Social Thinking Guidebook for Bright Teens and Young Adults* by Michelle Garcia Winner and Pamela Crooke
- *The Autism-Friendly Guide to Periods* by Robyn Steward
- *The Awesome Autistic Go-To Guide: A Practical Handbook for Autistic Teens and Tweens* by Yenn Purkis and Tanya Masterman
- *The Reason I Jump: One Boy's Voice from the Silence of Autism* by Naoki Higashida
- *The Spectrum Girl's Survival Guide: How to Grow Up Awesome and Autistic* by Siena Castellon
- *Unique: What Autism Can Teach Us About Difference, Connection and Belonging* by Jodi Rodgers
- *Welcome to Consent: How to Say No, When to Say Yes, and Everything in Between* by Yumi Stynes and Melissa Kang

NOVELS WITH ND MAIN CHARACTERS
- *My Life As an Alphabet* by Barry Jonsberg
- *On the Edge of Gone* by Corinne Duyvis
- *Please Don't Hug Me* by Kay Kerr
- *Social Queue* by Kay Kerr
- *The Kiss Quotient* by Helen Hoang
- *Underdogs:* Books 1–3 by Chris Bonello

OUT OF THE BOX

EMPLOYMENT FOR ND TEENS AND YOUNG ADULTS

Aurora Neuroinclusion Program helps autistic people or those with ADHD begin and progress a career in the Australian Public Service. (www.employforability.com.au/aurora/)

Australian Spatial Analytics is a not-for-profit social enterprise providing professional data services and Geospatial and Digital Engineering careers for young neurodivergent adults. (www.asanalytics.com.au)

auticon is an autistic-majority company which integrates their technology consultants into client organisations and provide inclusion and technology solutions for organisations looking to achieve their diversity goals. (www.auticon.com/au)

DXC Dandelion Program connects ND people with employment opportunities and helps workplaces also plug IT skills gaps. (www.dxc.com/au/en/about-us/social-impact-practice/dxc-dandelion-program)

'Neurodiversity, Equity, and Inclusion in MNCs' is an article published in *AIB Insights* (vol. 22, issue 3, 2022) that looks at ways neurodivergent employees are working within multinational corporations to create and promote awareness in global operating environments. (https://insights.aib.world/article/34627-neurodiversity-equity-and-inclusion-in-mncs)

Office for Autism is a dedicated office run by the Government of South Australia, where job seekers are able to seek help across a range of areas. For example, it includes workplace adjustments that

RESOURCES: FOR ND KIDS AND TEENS

employers might consider, as well as opportunities for autistic job seekers. (www.officeforautism.sa.gov.au)

Rise program was established by the former Victorian Department of Health and Human Services in 2017. It provides opportunities for autistic job seekers via alternative recruitment avenues. It uses half-day 'Discovery Days' to recruit employees, with the focus on their strengths and 'role-related capabilities'. (www.health.vic.gov.au/rise-program)

OTHER SUPPORT SERVICES

- 13YARN – 13 92 76 (www.13yarn.org.au)
- ADHD Foundation National Helpline – 1300 39 39 19 (www.adhdfoundation.org.au)
- Autism Connect – 1300 308 699 (www.amaze.org.au/autismconnect)
- Beyond Blue – 1300 22 4636 (www.beyondblue.org.au)
- headspace – 1800 650 890 (www.headspace.org.au)
- Kids Helpline – 1800 55 1800 (www.kidshelpline.com.au)
- Lifeline – 13 11 14 (www.lifeline.org.au)
- QLife – 1800 184 527 (www.qlife.org.au)

For the most up-to-date resource list and other *Out of the Box* companion resources, head to www.outoftheboxbook.com.au or scan the QR code for immediate access.

Welcome to Holland

Emily Perl Kingsley's 1987 essay has been reprinted below with the kind permission of the author. 'Welcome to Holland' provides an insight into her experience raising a disabled child that many parents find relatable.

I am often asked to describe the experience of raising a child with a disability – to try to help people who have not shared that unique experience to understand it, to imagine how it would feel. It's like this ...

When you're going to have a baby, it's like planning a fabulous vacation trip – to Italy. You buy a bunch of guide books and make your wonderful plans. The Coliseum. The Michelangelo David. The gondolas in Venice. You may learn some handy phrases in Italian. It's all very exciting.

After months of eager anticipation, the day finally arrives. You pack your bags and off you go. Several hours later, the plane lands. The flight attendant comes in and says, 'Welcome to Holland.'

'Holland?!?' you say. 'What do you mean Holland?? I signed up for Italy! I'm supposed to be in Italy. All my life I've dreamed of going to Italy.'

But there's been a change in the flight plan. They've landed in Holland and there you must stay.

The important thing is that they haven't taken you to a horrible, disgusting, filthy place, full of pestilence, famine and disease. It's just a different place.

So you must go out and buy new guide books. And you must learn a whole new language. And you will meet a whole new group of people you would never have met.

It's just a different place. It's slower-paced than Italy, less flashy than Italy. But after you've been there for a while and you catch your breath, you look around ... and you begin to notice that Holland has windmills ... and Holland has tulips. Holland even has Rembrandts.

But everyone you know is busy coming and going from Italy ... and they're all bragging about what a wonderful time they had there. And for the rest of your life, you will say 'Yes, that's where I was supposed to go. That's what I had planned.'

And the pain of that will never, ever, ever, ever go away ... because the loss of that dream is a very very significant loss.

But ... if you spend your life mourning the fact that you didn't get to Italy, you may never be free to enjoy the very special, the very lovely things ... about Holland.

— Emily Perl Kingsley
(C) 1987. All rights reserved.

ACKNOWLEDGEMENTS

WE STARTED THIS PROJECT WITH a blank piece of paper and so many questions. How do I know if my child is autistic? What's the best way to diagnose ADHD? Will my child be able to find a job? Date? Live on their own? Should they take medication? Get an ADHD coach? How can I help them find friends?

We don't have a real estimate of the number of neurodivergent children, or the power they hold, in our classrooms. Many children are not diagnosed. Others keep their diagnosis a secret because of a fear of judgement, and many have slipped through the cracks. It is our driving force to change that, and provide a clear and weed-free pathway for each neurodivergent child – and adult – to be their best self.

Our thank-you list could be as long as this book because almost 1300 parents and children told us their stories. You asked us how you could advocate for your child, and stand beside them while they navigate friendships and dating, and find employment. To every one of you, we hope we have listened with both ears and answered the questions you posed. Thanks for allowing us to join your journey in a bid to mute the discrimination in education and employment that too often dominates conversations around

ACKNOWLEDGEMENTS

autism and other brain variations. You encouraged us to look inside our classrooms to see how all children learn, and to better understand how teachers can access resources to deliver learning that triumphs. We are also appreciative of the help we received from the 600 teachers involved in our research, who answered our questions, in writing, close to midnight on a school night. With their combined input we hope these pages provide an easy-to-follow guide to navigate diagnosis and the challenges families are facing, and which will allow their kids to thrive. To everyone travelling that journey – not just the 2000 whose stories are the foundation of this book – we thank you.

We would have been lost without the experts – both neurodivergent and neurotypical – who helped us, and want to acknowledge both the generosity of their time and clinical wisdom. We could not have done this without the guiding hand of Kristy Forbes, Kate Foster, Emily Hammond, Kathy Hoopmann and Pip Williams.

Bronwyn Sutton, Sue Larkey and Justin Coulson answered our questions and provided unlimited professional advice, as did Mary Kaspar, Linda Graham, Mandira Hiremath, Yvette Anderson, Michael Bonning, Jodi Rodgers, Jenny Gribbin, Jasmine Parker, Cath Hakanson, Georgia Ostler, Ee-Lin Chang, Tamara Rosier, Aidan and Ross Greene. These kind and generous humans live across Australia and the globe, but saw the value in gifting the knowledge they've gained to help others.

Employers April Lea, Geoff Smith and Bodo Mann, and autistic workers Anthony and Harrison, made us understand the challenges of employment with startling clarity. Academics Leia Greenslade, Adam Guastella, Jessica Paynter, David Trembath and Jessica Hill opened our eyes to the challenges – but also the enormous hope – that exists in the field of research, and the need for lived experience in determining the path forward. Catherine Franklin reminded us, in her expert way, to always put the people we were writing about at the front and centre of our questions. There were many others too: Frank Brown and Deuk Rae Kim, Nicki Powell, Cam Russell and educators Jane Sullivan, Lisa Fife, Simone Kiprioti, Ann Edwards and Lisa Delaney. You will find their wisdom in these pages. Multiple Emmy Award-winner Emily Perl Kingsley and Emily Bourke, Australia's only politician whose portfolio is autism offered their help too. To all of you, this project only became alive as result of your kindness and engagement.

We owe a debt of gratitude to Andrew Whitehouse, Michelle Garnett, Wesley Turner and Tony Attwood. Not only did they suffer through long interviews and follow-up questions, but along with anonymous readers, they checked these pages, mindful of what we wanted to achieve and the need to help all those who are, or will, embark on a path not now considered the norm. Given the waiting lists to access any of these experts, we cannot thank them enough for the time – and guidance – they offered.

To our publisher Madonna Duffy, whose leadership was behind our choice of UQP as publisher; our ever-patient editor Jacqueline Blanchard, whose calm approach always ran counter to our deadline dramas; Christa Moffitt, who designed the cover; and the whole team at UQP, thanks for your support and hard work.

Finally, a heartfelt thanks to our families who stand by us, understanding how much better our communities can be, if we all – ND and NT – make an effort to understand the journey of those we walk beside.

INDEX

adults/older people with autism 250
advocating for your child's education, tips 100–1
after school years 187–209
    employment *see* employment
    post-school study *see* tertiary education
AI as a tool for ND children 101
AMAZE organisation 252
    tips for ND jobseekers 199–200
    website 252
Amazing Skills 256
Amazing Things Happen! video 264
Anderson, Yvette 22
anxiety 12
    co-occurrence with autism 11, 20
    The Brave Program 259
Asperger Syndrome (Asperger's)
    autism Level 1 29
    meaning ix
Assessment of Skills and Unsolved Problems (ASUP)
    online resource 139, 264
At Peace Parents 255
attachment trauma 62
Attention Deficit Disorder (ADD) ix
Attention Deficit Hyperactivity Disorder (ADHD)
    co-occurrence with autism 11, 240
    girls, under- or late diagnosis 2, 7, 14, 15

    meaning ix–x
    medication 22–3
    'naughty', being thought of as 8, 27, 125
    NDIS, exclusion from 228, 230, 243
    prevalence 2
    ways of presentation ix
Attwood, Professor Tony 9, 21, 102, 173, 185, 216, 254
Attwood & Garnett Events 254
autistic adolescents 56
    bullying, comments about 59
    friendships, comments on 45–6
    one friend, power of 65–6
Aurora Neuroinclusion Program 270
Australasian Society for Autism Research 240
Australian Spatial Analytics 195, 196, 270
Auticon Australia and New Zealand 201–2, 203, 270
    coaches, use of 203
autism
    ADHD, co-occurrence with 11, 240
    causes 239–41
    co-conditions 11, 240
    history of, diagnosis and treatments 250–1
    meaning x
    medical model, call to move away from 243
    other family members also having 20

autism (continued)
  premature infants and 240
  puberty and 21
  spectrum 29
  statistics around 250
  support, call to focus on 243
autism Level 1 10, 29
autism Level 2 29
autism Level 3 29
autistic high achievers, historical 191
autistic monotropism 217

Bargiela, Sarah 214
Barkley, Russell 254
belonging, importance of 53, 55
Birds and Bees 218, 253
  website 253
birthday parties 37–8
Black Dog Institute
  friendships, research as to importance 55
bluntness 39, 69
body language, difficulty reading 2, 211, 215
Bonning, Dr Michael 19, 26
Bonyhady, Professor Bruce 230
borderline personality disorder 20
Boulton, Kelsie 246
boundaries, communicating personal 71–2
Bourke, Emily 250
boys
  diagnosis, usually earlier than girls ix
  friendship and 78
  'naughty', labelled as 125
  Parenting Boys Peacefully website 256
  sextortion, target of 57
The Brave Program 259
BRAVING trust checklist 71
Brown, Dr Brene 71
bullied child, retaliation 135–6
bullying 47–50, 133
  dealing with, tips 50–1
  ND kids' vulnerability to 49
  online, via 56–8
  psychological effects of 59

Chang, Ee-Lin 63

change, difficulty managing 2, 13, 17
ChatGPT 101, 170
childhood disintegrative disorder (CDD) x
children
  6 or 7 years, recognising differences 35
  co-conditions with autism 10
    ADHD 11, 240
    common 11
    making identification difficult 11
    mental health conditions 247
    per centage of diagnoses, in 20
Collaborative and Proactive Solutions (CPS) 255–6
  model for classrooms 138–9
  website 256
Community Against Prejudice Towards Autistic People (CAPTAP) 256
connection, lack of 16
Coulson, Dr Justin 255
  Happy Families website 255
  three-point plan for separated parents 176–8
Covid, school experience during 11, 95

dating 210–12
  expectations of 219
  rejection 219
Davies, Allison 263
Delahooke, Mona 255
Delaney, Lisa 66, 67
Dent, Maggie 255
depression
  bullying, as a result of 59
  co-occurrence with autism 11, 20
diagnosis of autism
  access to support 17, 28
  awareness leading to increase in 19
  difficulties with 9
  lack of access to 25, 26, 144
  late 9, 15
  medical professionals involved in 17
  multidisciplinary approach 18
  national guidelines 17, 18
  quick tips for 31
  three-pronged approach 18

INDEX

Diagnostic and Statistical Manual of Mental Disorders (DSM-5) 29
diagnostic overshadowing x, 249
'disability', use of term 241–2
DivergAntz Collective 252
divorce
    more common where ND children 26–7, 174, 175–6
    three-point plan for separated parents 176–8
double empathy problem x, 42–3, 55–6, 217
drama classes, benefits 50
driving 220–2
    Assessing Fitness to Drive national standard 221
    licensing processes 222
    potential to drive assessment 221–2
drug and alcohol use 56
DXC Dandelion Program 270
dyscalculia x–xi, 3
dyslexia xi, 2, 194–5
dyspraxia xi, 2
    developmental coordination disorder (DCD) xi

early screening, research 246
early signs 10–17
    anxiety 12
    broadness of 11
    delayed speech 17
    disorganisation 12
    empathy, lack of 16
    food issues 12
    instructions, difficulty following 12
    lack of connection 16
    meltdowns, having 12, 126
    milestones, delayed 12
    neurotypical children, traits in 10
    parents, traits commonly noticed by 12
    ritualistic behaviours 12
    school refusal 12
    sensory challenges 12
    separation anxiety 12
    sleep issues 12
    social clues, missing 12, 40
    transition to school or high school, during 11
early supports 244–5
    Inklings Program for 6 to 18 months children 245
eating disorders 20
    autistic tweens and teens, occurrence among 11, 56
education system
    advocating for your child's education, tips 100–1
    autism focused schools 98
    Covid experience 11, 95
    modern, flexible learning methods 95
    national curriculum and set policies 94
    no best-practice policy as to neurodivergency 132
    school funding models 94
    teachers *see* teachers and educators
educational tools
    Assessment of Lagging Skills and Unsolved Problems (ALSUP) resource 139, 140
    Collaborative and Proactive Solutions (CPS) model for classrooms 138–9
Edwards, Dr Ann 99
Ehrlich, Casey 254–5
Elliott, Max 168
Elliott, Megan and Anthony 168
Emotion Sensation Feeling Wheel 265
emotions
    difficulty understanding other people's 2
    empathy, lack of 16
employment
    Aurora Neuroinclusion Program 270
    CV, preparing 199, 209
    digital economy 195–7
    employee assistance programs 193
    innovation skills 202
    interview process 198, 199–200, 209
    looking for 189–92
    resources for ND teens and young adults 270–1
    sensory environment 189, 197
    strengths of ND employees 192–5, 196, 201, 202, 209

employment (*continued*)
  tips for jobseekers 199–200, 209
  unemployment among people with autism 190–1
  what it provides in addition to money 190
eXceptional Learners 257
eye contact 8, 13, 43, 51

facial expressions
  difficulty understanding 2
families with neurodivergent members
  divorce, higher rate of 26–7
Family Planning Australia (FPA) 63
fidgeters 13
Fife, Lisa 80, 98–9, 107
financial literacy, planning for 208
Fisher, Naomi 256
flirting, understanding 64–5
Forbes, Kristy 28, 96–7, 133, 253
Foster, Kate 28, 29, 44, 191, 192
Franklin, Dr Catherine 249
Fraser, Jonelle 263
FreeSchool website 257
friendships, importance of 55–6
  Black Dog Institute research 55
  one friend, power of 65, 70, 81–2
friendships in high school 52–72
  belonging, no sense of 55
  boundaries, personal 71–2
  BRAVING checklist 71
  buddy systems 81
  bullying *see* bullying
  challenges faced, examples 54
  conversations, practising 70
  drug and alcohol use 56
  healthy friendships, recognising 71
  humour and 67–8
  listening skills, good 68–9
  loneliness at school 55
  marginalised groups, gravitation towards 56
  NT students, teaching about autism 74–5, 76, 83–4, 247–8
  one friend, power of 65, 70
  outside of school friendships 71, 170
  repairing, knowing how to 69–70
  role-playing conversations 68
  romantic relationships 61–5
  shared interests 66
  strengths, learning to manage 69
  team activities and clubs 50, 51, 66, 72
  time and energy, investing 72
  tips for helping with 70–1
  transition to, difficulties with 53
friendships in primary school 35–51
  acceptance and inclusion, model at home 51
  bullying and 47–50
  dealing with exclusion 46–7
  excluded, being 37, 38, 45–50
  'finding your tribe' 43
  good friendships, teach what they look like 51
  literal interpretation of everything 39
  outside school friends, focus on 51, 170
  parents' role 44–8
  positive feedback for showing friendship skills 42
  recognition of ability/personality differences 35–6
  stumbling blocks to making/keeping friends 39–41
  team activities and clubs 50, 51, 66, 72
  tenets of, teaching 42
  tips for helping with 51

Gadsby, Hannah 76
Garnett, Dr Michelle 15, 81, 88, 103–4, 114–15, 121–2, 128, 173, 216, 254
  Attwood & Garnett Events 254
  autistic adolescents 56
  books published by 253
Garvey, Billy 261, 263
gender, autistic teens questioning 11
gender dysphoria 20
general practitioners (GPs) 17, 19
genetics 18, 20, 239, 250
GingerCloud Foundation 168–9, 257

INDEX

girls
  anxiety or depression, impetus for seeking help 14
  ADHD, under- or late diagnosis 2, 7, 14, 15
  'mean girls' 48–9
  university, autism diagnosis at 14
glass child/children xi
  see siblings
Goon, Jasmine 184
government organisations, websites 259–260
Graham, Professor Linda 96, 118, 130, 138
Greene, Dr Ross 138, 139, 140, 254
Greenslade, Dr Leia 192–3, 242–3
Gribbin, Jenny 221
Guastella, Professor Adam 239, 244, 246

Hakanson, Cath 63, 212, 216, 259
  sex education 63–4
Hammond, Emily 30, 55–6, 118, 265
  NeuroWild 55, 265
Hansen, Mandy 15
Happy Families website 255
Hayden, Chloé 264
Heller, Theodor xii
Hey Sigmund website 255
high schoolers *see also* friendships in high school
  books for 268–9
  employment for ND teens and young adults 270
  Free School website 257
  Parental As Anything, Teens 256
  support helplines 271
Hill, Dr Jessica 24–5
Hiremath, Dr Mandira
  autism diagnosis 17–18, 238–9
  teaching primary school students about ND 247–8
history of diagnosis and treatments 250–1
homeschooling 92–4, 193
  disadvantages of 93
  increase in 92

  ND children 92–3
  reasons for 93
Hoopmann, Kathy 73–5
  The Essential Manual for Asperger Syndrome (ASD) in the Classroom 83
humour, sense of 7
  autism and 67–8

impulse control, lack of 13, 39, 54
in control, needing to be 39–40
Inklings Program 244–5
interpersonal skills, building 50
introverts 136–7

Josiah College 80, 98–9, 107
  model, acting as 99
Journal of Autism and Developmental Disorders 174

Kaspar, Dr Mary 48–9, 68–9, 88, 103, 174, 255
  friendships, importance of 55
  online resources for parents 176
  siblings of ND child 182
Kim, Deuk Rae (Dundee) 167–8
Kingsley, Emily Perl
  'Welcome to Holland' 172, 272–3
Kiprioti, Simone 98, 99, 107

label, differing views on 28
language, neuro-affirming 29–31
Larkey, Sue 77, 80, 103, 117, 122, 130, 170, 264
Lea, April 201
literal interpretations 39, 54
Lives in the Balance organisation 264
loneliness at school 55

management courses focusing on ND 249
Mandy, William 214
Mann, Bodo 201, 202, 203
masking xi, 1, 50
  romantic relationships and 62
  school, at 77–81, 137
Match Mate initiative 210–11

medication
  ADHD, for 22–3
  co-conditions, for 22, 23
  Spectrum Pharmacist 259
meltdowns 12, 126
  after school, at home 137
  lead up, signs 131
mental health
  co-conditions 246
  girls, levels in 78–9
  ND, higher risk of 246, 247
  NewAccess program 257
  supports for 247
'mentalising', encouraging 43, 50
Milton, Damian xiii, 55
Minds & Hearts 252–3
Mitchelson, Monique 15
Moeller, Dr Miriam 190–1
myths about neurodivergence 5–8

National Autism Indicators Report, 2021 262
National Disability Insurance Scheme (NDIS) xi, 225–30
  2020 review 226, 230
  ADHD, not included in 228, 230, 243
  appealing decisions 230–1
  applicants over 9 years 235
  application for, issues with 226, 227, 228, 233
  applications, tips for tackling 237
  children over 6, diagnosis required 233
  children under 6 years 232–3
  children with autism diagnosis, percentage 245
  conditions eligible for funding 227–8
  deficit-based model 225
  diagnosis, funding based on 230, 236
  early childhood partners 233
  eligibility meeting 234
  family impact statement 234
  'functional capacity', call to focus on 231, 236
  inconsistencies in funding 229, 236
  management of the plan offered 235
  navigating the system, difficulties 229, 232–7
  perspectives on 226–7
  professional reports 233–4
  regional clients 230
  'supporting evidence' 233–4
  supports available 234–5
  teacher, letter from 234
  therapy at school 236
National School Resourcing Board 232
'naughty', being thought of as 8, 27, 106, 118, 125, 133
neurodivergence
  challenges faced by people with 3
  early signs 10–17
  egocentricity 185
  percentage of school students with 1, 143–4
  range of conditions 3, 7, 80–1
neurodivergent (ND) children
  different presentations to different people 185
  labels and language used about 30–1
  meaning xi–xii
  students, refusal of any support 142
neurodivergent (ND) community 241
  research, influence on 242–3
neurodiversity, meaning xi–xii
'Neurodiversity, Equity and Inclusion in MNCs' 270
neurotypical (NT)
  children, and understanding autism 74–5, 76, 83–4
  meaning xii
NeuroWild 55, 265
NewAccess program 257
non-verbal, where 8

occupational therapists (OT) 17, 18, 19
Office for Autism 270–1
oppositional defiant disorder (ODD) xii, 3
organisations, websites 259–260
Ostler, Georgia 210, 211

INDEX

paediatricians 19
  children under 18, autism diagnosis by 17
Parental As Anything, Teens 256
parents
  acceptance and inclusion, model at home 51
  advocating for your child's education, tips 100–1
  barriers to community engagement 174
  burnout 185
  challenges of parenting ND children 173–4
  close relationships, impact of having ND child/children 174, 180
  dealing with exclusion of your child 46–7
  divorce more common where ND children 26–7, 174, 175–6
  exhaustion, constant 179, 180
  financial impact of having ND child/children 174, 180
  friendships, parents of ND child 45–50
  friendships, parents of NT child 45, 51
  future, worrying about 179, 181
  inconsistency in parenting NT and ND children 175
  judgment from others, dealing with 175
  mental health, impact of having ND child/children 174
  online resources 176
  pressure on 173–4
  problem areas facing 174
  refusal to seek assessment, where 109, 110, 142, 144
  resilience, teaching 47
  resources and experts 252–62
  stigma of ND child 27
  support, lack of identifying needs 174
  teachers, tips for building positive relationships with 152–4
  three-point plan for separated parents 176–8
  tips to cope 175, 186
Parker, Jasmine 199

pathological demand avoidance (PDA)
  increasingly common 21
  meaning xii, 21
Paul, Lisa 230
Paynter, Dr Jessica 240
peer connectedness, lack of 55
PEERS®
  social skills programs 257
Perler, Seth 264
pervasive developmental disorder (PDD) xii–xiii
pessimism and negativity 56
pharmacists 22
Planet Puberty 63, 258
podcasts for parents 261
Pokémon 161–3
pornography 60, 64, 65
Positive Partnerships organisation 258
  Online Planning Tool for parents 176
Powell, Nicki 226, 232, 254
premature infants 240
primary schoolers *see also* friendships in primary school
  books for 267–8
  Secret Agent Society programs 258
  support helplines 271
psychiatrist, autism diagnosis by 17
psychologists 17, 19, 22
puberty
  autism and 21
  Planet Puberty 63, 258
  preparing your child for 63
  Sex Ed Rescue 63, 212, 259
  sex education 63–4

Reframing Autism 258
research
  adults, about, lack of 250
  early screening 246
  early supports 244–5
  ND community influencing 242–3
  support and needs, call to focus on 243–4
resilience, teaching 47, 169, 170–1

resources
  Autism and ADHD organistaions and experts 252–4
  books for educators 266
  books for high-schoolers 268
  books for primary-schoolers 267
  books, podcasts, media and reports for parents 260–2
  educators, for 263–6
  employment for ND teens and young adults 270
  further learning for educators 264–266
  further learning and support for parents 256–60
  ND kids and teens, for 267–9
  parenting experts and organisations 254–6
  support helplines 271
Rise Program 271
ritualistic behaviours 12
Rodgers, Jodi 253
  dating role playing 219
  dating tips for autistic young adults 219–20
  Unique 218
romantic relationships 61–5
  autistic romance authors, reading books by 216
  dating role playing 219
  dating tips for autistic young adults 219–20
  feelings, acknowledging 62
  masking and 62
  NT and ND people, between 217
  sexual abuse, vulnerability of autistic young women 214
  talking about 216
Rosier, Dr Tamara 14, 204
  exclusion, dealing with 46–7
rule followers 13, 136
  reporting minor misdemeanours 41
Russell, Cam 168, 169

Safe Space Collective 201
sarcasm, failure to understand 40

school
  acknowledging and embracing ND 88–9
  bad, examples of 88
  education system *see* education system
  finding the right 87–8, 102–5
  gut instincts 103
  homeschooling *see* homeschooling
  learning support offered 103
  mainstream, failings or limitations of 88, 89, 90, 91, 95
  mapping the school campus 102
  openness to outside professionals 104
  punishments and rewards 113–16, 126–31, 132, 133
  supportive, examples of 91–2, 98–9, 133
  what to look for 104–5
  'whole school' 103
school avoidance 136 *see* school refusal
school culture
  academia and achievement 133–4
  Alex's story 124–5, 126–8
  inclusivity 134
  principal or head, set by 108–9, 128
school detentions 131
school dynamics 73–7
  buddy systems 81
  class sizes 117
  classrooms and sensory overload 118
  group work, challenges with 103
  masking in the playground 77–81
  multiple teachers and subjects, challenges with 77, 102
  no best-practice policy as to neurodivergency 132
  NT students and teachers, teaching about autism 74–5, 76, 83–4, 247–8
  NT students not understanding ND students 74–5
  pretending and masking 76
  punishments and rewards 113–16, 126–31, 132, 133
  suspensions 126, 129–31, 132, 134–5
  teachers not understanding ND students 76, 95–6, 97
  teachers, tips to assist ND students 96

INDEX

school refusal xii–xiii, 12, 96–7
school suspensions 126, 129–31, 132, 134–5
  damage and disconnection caused by 132, 135
Schore, Tosha 256
  Parenting Boys Peacefully website 256
Secret Agent Society
  programs for 8 to 12 year olds 258
self-advocacy, teaching 101
self-harm 59, 79
Seligman, Martin 69
sensory overload 2
  classrooms 118
  work situations 189, 197
separation anxiety 12, 129–30
Sex Ed Rescue 63, 212, 259
sex education 63
  consent, ensuring understanding of 213–14, 215
  early, importance of 212–13
  flirting, understanding 64–5
  masturbation 213
  resources, using 212–13
  Sex Ed Rescue 63, 212, 259
sextortion 57
sexual abuse
  autistic young women 214
Shore, Dr Stephen 2
shutting down 54, 136–7
siblings
  burnout 185
  empathetic stage 183–4
  glass child/children, known as 181
  impact of having a ND sibling on 181–3
  inconsistent treatment compared with ND sibling 181–2
  'it's not fair' stage 183
  psychological impacts on 182
Silove, Natalie 246
sleep disorders 20
Smith, Geoff 195, 200
social clues, missing 12, 40, 53, 54, 211
social justice, inflated sense of 13, 40

social media
  bullying via 56–8
  negative effects of 60
  sextortion 57
  tips in managing 61
social model of disability 96
Social Thinking website 259
Socially Speaking Game, The 265–66
Sparrow, Rebecca 256
Spectrum Pharmacist 259
speech, delayed 17
speech pathologists 17, 18, 19
sports programs
  GingerCloud Foundation 168–9, 257
stand-up comedians 191–2
status in a group 41
Steward, Robyn 214
stimming xiii, 8, 12, 142
strengths, acknowledging and learning to manage 69
Students with disability government website 265
substance abuse 20
suicidality 79
suicide, higher risk of 79, 247
Sutton, Dr Bronwyn 9, 15–16, 18, 173, 253
  advocating for a child's education, 100–1
  quick tips for diagnosis 31
Sydney Child Neurodevelopment Research Registry 246

Tajiri, Satoshi 162
Talking About Autism toolkit 266
Taylor, Ben 202–3
teachers and educators
  bad treatment of ND students 114–16
  burn-out 117
  good engagement with ND students 110–13
  handover with previous teacher 122
  identification of neurodivergence 15–16
  lack of training about ND 95–6, 97, 109, 114, 117
  ND students, not understanding 76, 95–6, 97

teachers and educators (*continued*)
  ND themselves, where 121–2
  over-worked, under-resourced and under-valued 117
  parents, working with 123
  punishments and rewards 113–16, 126–31, 132, 133
  relationship with students 107, 122
  resources 263–6
  reward systems 114
  teaching about ND 74–5, 76, 83–4, 232
  time, resources and support issues 108
  tips to assist ND students 96, 119–21
  trust, relationships of 107
  university education, inclusion of neurodivergency training 117–18
teachers' perspective
  challenges teachers face 143, 147–50, 155–6
  difficult parents, dealing with 154, 156
  parents' refusal to seek assessment 109, 110, 142, 144, 146
  positive impacts of ND students 150–2
  preparation involved in utilising support people 156
  professional development to teach ND students 145
  research at teacher's expense, and in own time 146
  supporting a ND child when family will not seek diagnosis 154
  under-valued, feeling 156
  undiagnosed ND, but exhibiting traits of 144
  violent ND students, managing 155
  what they want parents to know 157–8
teams and clubs
  benefits 50, 51, 66, 163–4, 171
  connections, helping to build 163, 164
  friendships outside school 170
  mentor figures 67, 165–7
  structured activities 169–70
  team sports, benefits 165
  tips for joining in 171

tertiary education
  advocacy for supports at institutions 206
  challenges facing students 206–8
  planning for 208
theory of mind concept xiii, 65, 184–5, 217
therapists 21–5
  animal-assisted 24–5
  canine therapy 24
  equine therapy 21, 24, 167
  lack of access to 25, 144
  music therapy 21
Tourette Syndrome xiii, 3, 20
Trembath, Professor David 242
Turner, Dr Wesley 22, 42, 184, 214, 252–3
  bullying, ND vulnerability to 49
  repairing friendships 69–70
  romantic relationships, comments on 62
  social media, comments on 60–1

unemployment among people with autism 190–1

vaccinations 241
videos (media) for parents 262

'Welcome to Holland', essay 272–3
Whitehouse, Professor Andrew 18, 95, 231–2, 240, 255
  Inklings Program 244–5
Williams, Pip 194–5

Yellow Ladybugs 146, 253
Young, Karen 255

Zimmerman, Dr David 252–3
Zones of Regulation framework 120, 124–5

www.ingramcontent.com/pod-product-compliance
Ingram Content Group UK Ltd.
Pitfield, Milton Keynes, MK11 3LW, UK
UKHW021314180426
11947UKWH00015B/1222